LIFE, SEX, AND PROSTATE CANCER SURGERY

LIFE, SEX, AND PROSTATE CANCER SURGERY

HOW ONE MAN HEALED AND WAS MADE WHOLE

John C. Hallenborg

Foreword by Fred S. Kuyt, M.D.

PRAEGER
An Imprint of ABC-CLIO, LLC

ABC CLIO

Santa Barbara, California • Denver, Colorado • Oxford, England

Library of Congress Cataloging-in-Publication Data

Hallenborg, John C.
Life, sex, and prostate cancer surgery : how one man healed and was made whole / John C. Hallenborg ; foreword by Fred S. Kuyt.
p. cm.
Includes bibliographical references and index.
ISBN 978-0-275-98135-8 (hardcopy : alk. paper) — ISBN 978-0-313-38148-5 (ebook) 1. Hallenborg, John C.—Health. 2. Prostate—Cancer—Patients—United States—Biography. I. Title.
RC280.P7H347 2009
362.196'994630092—dc22
[B] 2009018145

13 12 11 10 09 1 2 3 4 5

This book is also available on the World Wide Web as an eBook.
Visit www.abc-clio.com for details.

ABC-CLIO, LLC
130 Cremona Drive, P.O. Box 1911
Santa Barbara, California 93116-1911

This book is printed on acid-free paper ∞
Manufactured in the United States of America

For Debbie

Health alone is victory!

—Thomas Carlyle

CONTENTS

FOREWORD: A HANDS-ON LIFE

In choosing urology as a specialty, my goal was to put my hands where they would do the most good, helping men and women overcome maladies of an intimate nature. In addressing men's illnesses, prostate cancer looms as one of the most deadly. In treating the disease over a long career, I have worked with hundreds of men to give them a brighter future. My career has been very rewarding. The field of urology embodies so many lessons in human nature, man's insecurities and victories, our natural desire to procreate and recreate, and our need to grow old gracefully and comfortably.

With my career choice, to be blunt and clear, I became Fred the plumber of the lower human abdomen, unclogging pipes; relieving pressure, burning discomfort and pain; and often reconfiguring and rigging up an alternative way for better blood and urine flow. However, there are instances where the fix is life changing, because the problem threatens to destroy the patient. In addition to the surgery itself, my job is to convey to patients the importance of the task without creating a sense of a dark cloud cover. Hope must be maintained. In diagnosing illnesses, I inform my fellow human beings about all the possible ways problems can be solved according to the specific requirements of that person's way of feeling and thinking. Thus, this element of my profession is unique for each patient. There is no focused training for it. I must look people square in the eye and transmit the good news as well as the bad news, assuring my patients that no matter what, I will be with them until the job is done and the fine tuning is complete. The celebration will simply be the rest of their life, and what they choose to do with it.

As for prostate cancer, who would think that a small cellular defect within an organ the size of a walnut, located in parts unknown, yet close indeed to the family jewels both anatomically and functionally, could cause such havoc? How do you get to parts unknown? How do you know if all of those cellular defects have been removed? The real question my prostate cancer patients ask themselves is some version of: "Will I be a whole man again, once the prostate gland is extricated and the repair is complete?"

That question was in the forefront of my patient John's mind between the time of his diagnosis and his surgery. John was going to be a tough nut to crack. A smile required a real reason to cause that familiar configuration of dour lips and face to change; he had not yet found a way to reach internal biochemical equilibrium. He had no tolerance for platitudes or clichés. He was straightforward and commanded straightforward honesty, but preferred it with grace and dignity. His intelligence could not be avoided, nor could his understanding of the human condition be separated from what he was about to hear. He was told at the local health clinic that, at age 46, it was not a bad idea to get a baseline PSA (a measure of Prostate Specific Antigen, which can signal health or disorder). After all, those three letters were the talk of the nation, as more and more male celebrities made it known that they had prostate cancer. Taboos against discussing it had fallen. John had the wisdom to listen to the person who knew more than he did on this topic. I could tell he did not take instruction well. Yet his uncle had had the surgery in his 70s, and had lived another 15 years after his diagnosis and subsequent treatment of prostate cancer.

I had John's blood tested and his PSA came back at 6.2. Any result north of 4.0 is abnormal, so there was cause for concern. He did not have any signs of prostate infection, something that could falsely elevate this number, nor had he engaged in one of life's primary pleasures within 24 hours prior to having his blood drawn. There was no explaining away the elevated blood value of John's prostatic specific antigen, a protein produced exclusively by the prostate gland. As men who looked straight ahead, neither of us equivocated about the importance of discovering the naked truth. Therefore, we embarked upon a journey of many miles. This book is a key part of the journey I share with John.

Once it becomes imperative to determine if a guy does indeed have prostate cancer, it is time for a biopsy. Most patients hear the following when they are biopsied: "Please roll onto your left side and assume the fetal position. Move a little closer to the edge; trying to relax is your option, but breathing slowly and regularly will help . . . No, this is not my finger, it's longer, it's the ultrasound probe. When you hear the click, you might jump a bit, but please remain on the table." I try to talk my way through every intimate examination and procedure, as this approach calms most patients (the ones who are conscious; in surgery they are not) when I take things step by verbal step. After the first biopsy core is taken from the prostate gland, you know what to expect and you become a little less apprehensive. Back in 1999, I sent men like John to another specialist for the biopsy; today, I perform them in my office. When I saw John after his biopsy, I asked him how he was doing, but he just said we were in this thing together. John had my personal cell phone number in case questions popped up and he needed quick reassurances.

"Hello John, it's Fred. How are you feeling today? Good. Well, I do have some good news and a bit of bad news. One of the six cores did demonstrate a small cluster of cancer cells, not too aggressive, but not to be ignored. It looks as if we've caught it early in its inception. That's obviously the good news. You will be all right, John. We have many choices on how to approach this problem, so why don't you come in as soon as possible? Please ask Debbie to come with you; she'll remember what you don't."

Knowing that John did not deal well with uncertainty, I knew he would be much better off not having to guess at what his post treatment PSA values meant. If you choose a treatment other than surgery when the cancer is confined to the gland, you are likely to have PSA values that fluctuate above zero from time to time. This would have driven John crazy as he wondered what was going on in his body all the time. He was not afraid of surgery, and was clearly the type of person who wanted the "unwelcome guest" removed from the party. We reviewed less invasive ways to cure him, but John's nature dictated what to him was the most definitive approach. With the surgery, if all went well, the cancer would be in one place, off to a lab, and John in another, off to live his life. With internal or external radiation, the gland would remain inside of him, as would any cancer cells still lingering after treatment. Although the statistics were comparable, an uneven postsurgical future seemed to be too uncertain for John's personality.

Again, to put it into simple terms that everyone can understand, I have been cleaning, bending, and reconfiguring human urinary pipes for nearly 27 years. My training and practice have always emphasized urologic oncology, of which prostate cancer is by far the most common condition within that subspecialty of the subspecialty. I have attended and participated in more than three dozen local, national, and international conferences on prostate cancer, and diagnosed more than 1,300 men age 42 and over with the disease. Over that same time, I have performed and/or participated in more than 1,000 radical prostatectomies in selected patients ranging up to 78 years of age.

As in all areas of medical treatment, one technique has a tendency to give way to another. In the office, we now perform radical prostatectomies using the highly touted robotically assisted laparoscopic method. (This advance has occurred thanks to my very talented and much more recently trained associate.) The major advantage of this procedure is that blood loss is almost always kept to a minimum and the need for blood transfusion is extremely rare, rather than commonplace as it is with the "open" RRPPLND (radical retro-pubic prostatectomy with pelvic lymph node dissection). John describes both procedures in detail in this book.

Of the surgical candidates, nearly all of whom were well selected for cure, approximately 60 percent were cured after the first go-round with surgery alone, and 75 percent were cured after the initial pathology report from surgery indicated questionable margins and that using adjunctive radiation therapy would be necessary to affect a cure. The other 25 percent would require treatment with testosterone ablation therapy.

The toughest cases are of course the ones that are incurable at the time of initial presentation. I recall a 44-year-old gentleman, as humble and kind as could be, intelligent, thoughtful, a family man, an aficionado of healthy living. His PSA was only 1.9, within the "normal" range, but he had a strong family history of prostate cancer. His biopsies showed 9 out of 22 biopsy cores to be positive with adenocarcinoma of the prostate gland. This man's cancer had escaped the gland, which always carries negative complications of varying severity. Indeed, his high score indicated aggressive disease, and when the bone scan was done and showed widespread metastatic disease, many hearts were broken. He just recently lost his battle after five years of radiation, hormone ablation, chemotherapy, plus alternative care.

Another very tough case involved a 56-year-old hypochondriac, very sincere and concerned, who sought four different opinions before making his treatment choice. His clinical situation dictated that he was very likely to be cured. Indeed, six years after an apparently perfect technical operation, he was biochemically negative for prostate cancer, still using thick protective pads every day for urinary incontinence, and incapable of and uncaring about sexual activity. He felt that he had made the wrong choice for him, and that we had won the battle but lost the war. Post-op depression set in, and he has not yet found a way out of it.

Yet the sweet victories far outnumber those frustrating and devastating events. Among these are the men who present with a PSA value in the high teens or low 20s whose PSA numbers revert to normal <4.0 values after an infection is treated with antibiotics, and those men who show no biochemical recurrence of prostate cancer after 10 years, who can happily consummate romance, and who do not require any form of protective garment for incontinence. Still, when all is said and done, the success of the treatment is proportionate to the priorities of the individual men who have undergone treatment. I have not so infrequently encountered men who are cured and who are continent, but have indeed lost the ability to have spontaneous erections without the use of supportive measures. They literally feel that their lives are over and that their manhood is essentially nonexistent. On the other hand, there are those who are eternally grateful for their second chance in life and feel that being alive is all they would have hoped for. I must say I have encountered significant numbers of men like this, though they are in the minority. So explaining and considering the quality of life issues, according to each individual's priorities and personality, is just as important as the treatment options in determining success of the outcome.

This last group includes men who are fortunate to muster a great attitude. "All right! OK! I survived! I've been told that I'm cured! I'm still alive to smell the roses and enjoy the company of my loved ones, and I only missed seven days of work! That hideous rubber tube they call a Foley is no longer stuck inside that sensitive inner part of my 'member.' Wow! What's that warm feeling coming down my leg? Why did this happen as soon as I felt a burning sensation at the tip of my penis?" Some guys are blessed with the ability to stay upbeat, come what may.

So there you are, three months after surgery, sore from Kegel exercises, still wearing one or two protective pads per day and opting for only black or dark blue trousers. Perhaps you're simply depressed about having to take Vitamin V in order to obtain a burrito-like erection and a four-Motrin headache. Fair enough, but the alternatives are worse.

Once the high of life-positive victory subsides, there is always some form of aftermath. In 5–10 percent of postsurgical radical prostatectomy patients, there is urinary incontinence of varying degrees. Amongst these men, almost all will feel the need to wear a protective pad, sometimes temporarily and sometimes permanently. Fortunately, a relatively minor procedure can correct this form of incontinence. On the other side of the coin, more than 90 percent of postsurgical radical prostatectomy patients are completely continent of urine with the exception of one tiny caveat; without exception, almost all men will have slight stress urinary incontinence. That means that when your bladder is full, the way it is after drinking a few martinis or beers, when you cough or sneeze or strain to lift or bend, small amounts of urine will squirt out involuntarily. So be sure to pee before drinking alcohol, and do not wait until your urge to void is severe. Otherwise, you will just have to live with this minor inconvenience. Most men can and do live that way without too much ado.

As for sexual function after your RRPPLND, you have to be prepared for the fact that it will not be the same. In fact, it can be quite different yet, fortunately, often still satisfying. This does require some serious attitude adjustment. Since the source of semen has been removed along with your cancer-containing walnut, orgasm will be dry, unless you have the rare distinction, like John, of occasionally ejaculating some urine instead. The rule of thumb, or of the penis for that matter, is that if you are unequivocally potent prior to surgery—and this should be according to the female partner and not according to the wishful male's perception—and if both erectile nerves were spared, then after surgery there is a 70 percent chance of retaining sexual potency adequate for vaginal penetration.

Some men, let's say most men, will nonetheless require prophylactic erectile conditioning with Viagra intake. Some men will require this in conjunction with suction devices, therapy or low-dose penile injection therapy. Some men will always require one of the alternative supportive measures in order to consummate romance. Others, especially those with presurgical erectile dysfunction of varying degrees, men with atherosclerotic vascular disease, long-standing high blood pressure or diabetes, men with a significant smoking history of greater than two packs per day, or those men in whom only one nerve could be spared due to the extent of their disease, erectile function will not be possible without penile implantation. Some men, however, simply do not care enough to deal with this part of the aftermath. In any event, it all requires openness and a willingness to pursue the supportive measures, if needed, to resume an acceptable quality of life, albeit a changed one. A supportive partner is at the top of the list amongst the most critical ingredients in determining the success of rehabilitative therapy.

I must emphasize with great enthusiasm that a diagnosis of prostate cancer today carries a vastly improved prognosis from what it did as recently as 10 years ago. Methods of earlier detection, improvements in minimally invasive surgical techniques and instrumentation, improvement in the delivery systems of both internal and external radiation therapy, are all part of the ongoing advancement in treating prostate cancer.

Current research in the field of prostate cancer is pursuing the formulation of radio-sensitizing substances that render prostate cancer more vulnerable to selective killing effects. Current research is also pursuing the preemptive effects of gene therapy on preventing prostate cancer tumor growth, as well as identifying metabolites found in the urine that can predict the onset of prostate cancer in particularly aggressive forms of disease. All of these discoveries-in-progress will continue to improve the prognosis of prostate cancer in the future.

What follows here is an interesting, enlightening, honest read whose goal is to reach a large and growing male population needing and seeking front-line debriefing; it will help you cope, make decisions that are best suited for you as an individual, and make you feel far less alone. Battle on!

—Fred S. Kuyt, M.D.

ACKNOWLEDGMENTS

Among the remarkable people in my life, the following individuals have helped to build bridges from one growth phase to the next. I am grateful to you all, as well as to Alcoholics Anonymous: the late Olga Basset; the late Kathleen D. Casey; the late Eliot "Kidd" Cohen; Terry "TD" Davis; Ausbert DeArce; Ami and Brent Ducoing; Alexandra, my sister Ingrid, Matthew, and Ron Durham; T. J. Elliott; Annette Garner; Dennis Goddard; Charles Goldman; Kirk Hallam; my brother Steven Hallenborg and his family; the extended Hallenborg family; George Hambrick, MD; Maddy and Chuck Herman; Francis Hines; James Jackson, PhD; Jim Jones; Karen Johnson; Burt Kearns; Siranoush Kevorkian, MD; Tom Levin; Thornton Lewis; Gregg Miller, PhD; Tom Mahoney; Eric Manikowski; the Manikowski family; Nancy Moro; Byron Nilsson; Regina and Frank Ollari; Denise Quaglia; Kim Shamsky; Ted Shuttleworth; Melinda Tennison; Eleanor Whitledge; Virginia Wiese.

Special Acknowledgments

At critical times, when I needed support the most, these individuals stepped up. They will forever hold a special place in my heart. My humblest thanks to you: Jesi Burch; the late L. Nicholas Deane; Jillian Gross; my mother, the late Ida Hallenborg; Fred S. Kuyt, MD; Paula Manikowski; David Milch; E. Patrick Miller; Thomas Boyd Nash; Mike Vietro.

In Memory

Of my late father, Walter S. Hallenborg, who did the best he could with the tools he had.

INTRODUCTION

In 1999, I was diagnosed with prostate cancer, as were more than 200,000 other American men. With no cure in sight 10 years later, men mostly 50 and older face this potentially fatal disease with varying degrees of calm or panic. Unusually, I was only 46 years old when I chose to undergo a radical prostatectomy (RP) in October 1999. This choice was radical indeed, as it involves cutting the entire prostate gland out of the body through the frontal groin area, while rerouting the urinary and sexual plumbing and attendant blood vessels. My other options at that time were wait and see (never an approach for the impatient), having strongly radioactive seeds implanted in or near the gland, or undergoing periodic radiation treatments focused on the gland via beam techniques, perhaps in tandem with hormone therapy. Since my ordeal, another method employing laparoscopy is evolving in the United States to become standard procedure in more affluent regions. This procedure entails a tiny camera and cutting tools to excise the cancer. A version championed in France has the camera and tools going into the penile opening while, more commonly in the United States, five small incisions are made in the abdomen and the implements are guided in accordingly.

By nature, I am an information junkie. Once interested in a medical issue, I become obsessed to know all there is to know about it, up to the point where I'd need a medical degree to know more. This didn't begin when I was diagnosed with the disease; I can quickly become obsessive about information gathering on any subject if it holds my interest. It is all I can do after watching an episode of *House* to keep from running to the computer and spending hours researching the rare disease-of-the-week as profiled on that very clever TV show.

So mere hours after my diagnosis, I set out to get my hands on every book in print about prostate cancer, along with medical tomes about the molecular science of cancer. There were plenty of good books about the disease and its treatments, yet I found little about what it is like from a psychological point of view to experience the successive shocks of diagnosis, treatment and aftermath. As my surgery date approached, and later, after surgery, I thought more and more about this void in information, which led to what I have been told is a graphic article I wrote for the *Washington Post* in the summer of 2001. As the paper published my e-mail address along with the 1,500-word version of my story, hundreds of e-mails poured in from around the world, all but one thanking me for my candor and specificity. The one unhappy respondent was upset that I described sexual behavior out of wedlock. Heaven forefend. One surprising element in the e-mails was that a third of the respondents were women, thanking me for prompting a dialog with their pre-op or post-op husbands or boyfriends. Some of these e-mails are reprinted in Chapter 7.

This strong response was what I had hoped for, and with this book, an expanded version of the article, I hope to extend the ongoing dialogue into as many prostate cancer-affected homes as possible, both in the United States and abroad. I have tried to bring to this recovery narrative the writer's tools I have honed over 30 years as a writing professional, striving to balance objective and subjective perspectives in order to most benefit readers. Fair warning, however. I am an incurable wiseass, so if you are easily embarrassed or offended by blunt, descriptive language about sexual and medical matters, you may have to wait for a book written by the offended sanctimonious *Post* reader to gain the whitewashed knowledge he might impart. Sex to me is fun, and I have no hang-ups about discussing it. Chalk that up to my emergence from a household with northern European roots.

I chose to have the cancer cut out for a number of reasons, but foremost was the desire to make it separate from me, to "put it in a jar," as Dr. Bob Milch advised me. He had had the surgery years earlier. The alternatives involving radiation came with a risk I found unacceptable. Once the tissue in the affected area is irradiated, if the cancer flares up again, one cannot then choose surgery, as the irradiated tissue will not heal. One would simply bleed out. However, I can understand why other men choose alternative forms of treatment, and I sincerely hope representatives from those camps write books to share their experiences. I choose not to speculate about cancer treatment roads I have not personally taken.

If you are about to undergo a radical prostatectomy, or if you have recently undergone the procedure and you want to know what it feels like to recover from it over the course of nearly 10 years, this book is for you. This story is also for you if you are the wife or significant other of a man facing the procedure and its aftermath. Men in Western culture have been indoctrinated with a set of arbitrary "tough guy" rules that include near-silence in the context of trauma and physical or psychological pain. Adhering to these societal norms can make recovery much more difficult. These social norms, a drum I will beat repeatedly, are a bunch of nonsense, useful at the front lines in war and nowhere else. Please understand that the procedure requires recovery measured in years; it can be arduous and requires patience if one is to not unravel psychically. Still, the worst of it is measured in weeks, so do not despair. If your cancer has escaped the prostate capsule, you are in for a longer haul than I experienced. All the more reason to seek active treatment and proper follow-up. If this book was written in opposition to anything, it is to the watchful waiting that some doctors condone.

Some forms of disease-related suffering emerge out of bad choices, such as suffering in stoic silence as one's loved ones wring their hands wondering what they can do to make your recovery easier. This is undoubtedly a common scenario in America, as many communications with fellow prostate cancer patients have taught me. Some aspects of this experience are common to us all and others are unique to the individual. Hence my dual approach: objective and subjective, facts and feelings.

A quick example: shortly after removing the catheter and urinary bag I had worn for a few weeks following the surgical procedure, I came down with a cold; this was on top of the fact that my scrotum had swelled to the size of a grapefruit. I prepared some tea and drank it down. It went through my rerouted plumbing and down my leg before I made it out of the kitchen. Duly warned, you think you are ready for these episodes of physical disempowerment, yet they are always unsettling. Early on after surgery, incontinence was complete and very alarming, and some men in these circumstances never regain good urinary control. Such was one of many thoughts marching around in the back of my mind. It felt like I was pouring the tea down a three-foot hose attached to my mouth that emptied onto my leg. Thoughts included, Would I be wearing a diaper forever? What woman would put up with that?

If as a man you are comfortable speaking openly about your feelings, you will have a much easier time with the recovery process, as it will take months to restore you to something approaching your former physical self. Your mental self, well, that's a more complicated matter. As a youth, I was well taught to suppress my feelings. If it hurts, walk it off, and get on with it. Many American men will identify with that. As one result, I had a tougher time of it than if I hadn't bought into this very negative American tradition, inherited from our staid Anglo-Saxon forebears. Men in our culture are not sufficiently trained to distinguish between personal toughness and stubborn stupidity.

And then there are communications with women. Oh, how I wish things between men and women were different when it comes to communication! Though I may have been in several long relationships, and although I speak only for myself, I suspect most men would begrudgingly agree that talk is necessary to maintain healthy relationships. Generally, I put off conversation because it's too much work to pierce the veils of politeness and sociability. I have particular areas in which

I can be very lazy, and this is one of them. Sometimes I look back fondly on the few times I lived alone. Days would pass when no speech was required. I would hunker down with cereal and Stouffer's microwavable meals and write, write, write, nap, write, write, write some more. Of course, relentless hormones would accumulate and I would need to take care of that, one way or another. Well into my 40s, my libido was still raging, dictating much of my thoughts and behavior. Do I prefer ideas to people? Depends on which day you ask me, but there are times when ideas compel my focus more readily. When I am plugged in to work, this is the case, as writing is for the most part a solitary business. Relationships are put on the back burner to simmer, get overcooked, scalded, what have you. And yet, my love for those who are close to me knows few bounds in terms of depth of feeling. The joy is great, the disappointments excruciating.

My hope is that men will give themselves the gift of good communication if it does not come naturally, as recovering from prostate surgery is sure to derail a guy from the routine tracks of thoughts and feelings of everyday life. Your love partner and friends can help you get back on track, so please, do not be too proud or "tough." Let people help you. Let me tell you about a strapping ex-Marine, 65 or so to whom I tried to give advice. Though he'd been diagnosed with prostate cancer, he did not have any symptoms. This is common, as prostate cancer is often a painless killer until it is too late to cure it. This tough guy refused to believe there was anything wrong with him until he felt pain in his back. He is deceased today, from prostate cancer left untreated for too long. He died hard. As you have probably heard, early detection can save your life. It saved mine.

So when wonderful Dr. Fred Kuyt confirmed that I had cancer, I commenced reading. I am a natural writer and reader, with very little formal education. I hated school from age seven on, as I found academic environments plodding and constricting. It has been suggested I buy a Harley and have Born To Read tattooed on my back, but a gang of such inclination would be too circumspect to have much cultural impact. The flip side is, I have a tendency to hide in books when I should be communicating with others one-to-one or in group settings. My prostate cancer ordeal taught me to open up with people, and more often. There is no substitute for human contact, and when cornered by the peculiar anxiety and frustration associated with temporary incontinence, temporary impotence and a selection of other debilitations, I learned to speak up and ask for help and support. I hope everyone who reads this has others they can turn to, as it may make the difference between a smooth recovery and a rocky trip through an especially exasperating purgatory. If these pages help make things go more smoothly for some men and their loved ones, then I've done what I set out to do. *Avanti!*

—John C. Hallenborg
Redondo Beach, California, May 9, 2009

One

BACK STORY

Until I was diagnosed with prostate cancer, I never reflected much on how rewarding middle age had been for me. Yet I carried around a sense of vulnerable gratitude that appeared to be dour determination. Any feelings of self-acceptance I possess today, only occasionally disturbed, are in vivid contrast to the self-loathing hell that was my youth, teens and twenties. Consistent mood swings between mild anxiety and something akin to serenity have been hard won. Though I was a happy kid up to age seven, after that I was chronically angry and clinically depressed until age 50. Forty-three years of considerable psychic distance from even my closest friends and lovers did not promote happiness, which eludes me still. But at present I enjoy long stretches of contentment, with precious detours into joy. This is the reward for positive risk-taking, the most important behavior for an adult of an artistic temperament. I am no stranger to negative risk-taking, and continue to pay for past bouts of desperate behavior.

Despite what should be a weak psychological foundation for recovering from serious illness, I have done so successfully several times. Patting myself on the back for surviving cancer, bleeding ulcers, alcoholism and chronic depression may seem to be out of line, but so be it. These facts of my medical history are germane to my story, just as my readers' health is inextricable from their lives. The point is, I got through it all and I am now healthy and prepared to tell the tale. Feeling better now than I ever have before, I have no sense of the decline that comes with aging, not yet, anyway. A few creaky moments in the mornings at age 56, but that's about it.

I was conceived in the spring of 1952, in a small hotel in Finland, where my parents had gone to help a secret group of Europeans who were intent on overthrowing

Stalin's regime and installing true socialist leadership. Failing that, they returned to the States. I was born in a windblown shack on a frozen lake in Minnesota. My father had long been a frozen-lake fisherman, selling his lake trout catches to restaurants in St. Paul and Minneapolis. When my mother went into labor, she dutifully drove to the remote lake to give birth to me as part of Viking tradition. It was minus 30 degrees Fahrenheit, the moon high in a deep indigo sky, as she waddled across the ice to the tiny hut. My dad arranged the blankets that had been passed down for 15 generations. He urged my mom on, chanting in a lost Swedish dialect. At 1:44 A.M. on January 29, 1953, by candlelight, I popped out, screaming bloody murder. My dad cut the cord with a chop from an 11th-century iron hatchet and performed a Norse pagan ritual. I found my place in the mortal coil.

Take Two. Some of you bought into that windswept scenario. Thank you for your romantic inclinations. The truth is more mundane, as it generally is, but there are special moments. Early in my life, my mom was a homemaker and had been a brilliant swimmer, qualifying for the Olympics. She didn't go because she had to work to help support her family as, in July 1927, her Argentinean (German and French) immigrant father had hung himself in their New York City tenement basement when she was three months old. She never knew her father had killed himself so soon after her birth, which is just as well. Yet she turned out to be a normal, very bright girl. Her name was Ida Basset, and her sisters were Florence and Anita; I've always loved old-school names like that. In 1953, at 27, my mom looked much like a swollen, blonde Rita Hayworth when I was born in New York Hospital at the time and date mentioned above. My father, Walter S. Hallenborg, was a 30-year-old teacher, tall and skinny, and a gifted actor and singer. He had been a cut-up corporal and radioman in the Army Air Corps during WWII, honing his considerable acting skills in service productions. My mom and dad met at a Lutheran church social. They married and moved into an apartment on New York's Upper East Side. This was Yorktown, where many other immigrants' children of northern European descent had settled. Both of my parents were very left politically, socialists misplaced in America. My mother's mother, the widow Olga (Nana to me) Basset, a Finnish stoic of the Grant Wood school, lived with my parents until her death in 1983. She and my mom shared childcare duties. Shortly after my birth, their artsy friend Des wrote and recorded a song about me called "Big Blue Eyes." I have a copy of it somewhere. It never charted, although it made my mom and dad's Top 40.

When I was two, the family moved to Bethpage, Long Island, where my father taught junior high students and my mother kept house. My first clear memory is of taking all the pots out of the cupboard under the kitchen sink, banging and then arraying them on the floor and matching the correct tops to each pot. I thought I was doing everybody a favor, making my point in complete sentences. I recall a state of perfect confusion as my mother, responding to the charivari, insisted on undoing my fine work and returning the pots and tops to their respective locations, their natural union broken. The woman was surely insane, I decided, and I wailed to that effect unconvincingly. But with the pots and tops escapade, I had evinced a predisposition toward set theory, which when coupled with a prodigious memory and ability to synthesize, led to my becoming a writer, who learned by reading.

So at age three, I discovered books, and my intellectual fate was mostly sealed. I think my mom first read me *A Hole Is to Dig*, and that was it; a word monster was created. It wasn't long before I was reading *Curious George Flies a Kite* and the Dr. Seuss classics, my favorites of which were *McElligot's Pool* and *If I Ran the Zoo*. These books had wild creatures running amok, exposing the idea that our minds and artistic creations were not limited to the realm of reality, which continues to disappoint. A few years later, given my bleak personal reality, my imagination became an engine of solace and fantasy.

My early childhood entailed much analytical scrutiny. My father was a proud educator and I was his guinea pig to some degree, a fate not shared by my younger sister and brother after my father befriended the bottle for good. My old man was fascinated by every aspect of my early development. Early on he was very pleased by my precocious style, but as his alcoholism progressed, he came to resent it. At age eight or 10 or so I was given the standard IQ tests for kids and got all the answers correct, which triggered tougher tests usually reserved for military enlistees. After that I was treated as something of a freak.

I thought and spoke like an adult at a too-young age, playing with syntax and points of view, so much so that my Aunt Evelyn (Bowen, nee Hallenborg) thought I was possessed by a demon. I began to refer to myself in the third person as "He," as in: "He is sick today and will not be attending school." Then "he" became "John," as in "John is taking Maxie (my German Shepherd and best buddy) for a walk." Aspects of that obnoxious behavior linger today, as I like to amuse and get a rise out of people. I safely assess myself as a wiseass who in some key respects refuses to grow up. As a writer, it is important to easily access the layers of growth and experience that have accumulated. I can readily think and act like a 17-year-old if prompted. Yet, also, like a curious kid, today I must seek out fresh challenges, as boredom sets in easily. Exposed to ideas new or old, I learn very quickly and navigate the modern world with a well-worn awareness. Surprises and confusion are mostly the dubious province of others. I smile in irony, in defeat, in Indiana, and when in proximity to a gorgeous woman.

At around age six, I engaged my first girlfriend in stolen kisses on her doorstep. Patti had curly blonde hair coiffed by her mother, who loved my devilish comments. Patti's father, a mobbed-up general contractor, glowered at me when I came over for lunch. His mask of intimidation was all the warning I needed: Fathers protect their daughters from interlopers, no matter how young or well intended. Later I may allude to a theory not mine, namely: Obstacles plus excitement equals attraction. I wonder what happened to the guys who dated pretty Patti once she reached dating age. Better them than me.

By 1960, I was a restless seven-year-old in solid middle class circumstances, complete with a white picket fence, a big dog and a modest yard. The all-white neighborhood was as bourgeois as Beaver Cleaver's, an open-faced kid I thought was a jerk. As my father's drinking escalated, so did his raucous fights with my mother. One time when he was drunk, he drove a rental car way too fast to my relatives' house in Brooklyn, with me in the passenger seat next to him, as he ranted about his frustrations. All his life he'd wanted to be an actor full-time and not a teacher "on a hamster wheel," as he put it. He was a huge presence, a demigod to me, but my underlying belief, cultivated over the first six years of my happy existence, that he would protect me from harm, went out the window that day and forever. Things only got worse. Connecting these passive/aggressive concepts was an insidious, fomenting cynicism that clouded my subsequent judgment then, somewhat less so now.

Meanwhile, ostensibly happy neighbors mowed their lawns and got to know each other over the low fences meant to delineate New Deal property. There were barbecues, and trips to Coney Island and Jones Beach. I rode my Thunderjet bike and played with Maxie, a gift to me on my second birthday, and I felt something vague and powerful for my 14-year-old neighbor, a frowzy girl who improved the neighborhood by leaving her shirt open. I had to look, yet I didn't quite know why.

One fall day in 1960, while Nana watched over my infant brother, Steve, my mother and I walked my four-year-old sister, Ingrid, down the street to a young girl's birthday party, despite the imminent threat of Hurricane Donna. I wondered aloud why we would risk such an outing. My mother explained that the birthday girl was dying of cancer. This was my first exposure to the grave consequences of this disease in someone I knew, as in the '60s, a cancer diagnosis almost always meant a death sentence. The general C-word gloom factor back then was at least 10 times what it is today. I picked up on my mother's tone, which was consistent with the dire messages from other adults I had heard speak about the disease, or "the Big C," as they called it. I asked for an explanation and got a terse, circular one.

The hurricane blew over and the huge tree fallen in our yard was cut up for firewood. Neighbors grew a little closer, sharing stories with my parents, sometimes of a personal nature. Fascinated by anything that upset adults, as I determined there must be hidden substance there, I turned to my trusted *Encyclopedia Britannica* for answers about cancer. There were phrases about "uncontrolled cell growth," which I equated with growth in general, a process I was familiar with and had thought of as positive. Other matters soon distracted me, though, and I thought little about cancer until my teens.

When I was nine, in 1962, the six-member family moved to Connecticut, where my father landed a job as a junior high school principal in tony Greenwich. One afternoon a local truant put a knife to my throat and I didn't buckle. My dad took care of it, his last protective gesture toward me that I can recall. After a year of renting a house in the tick-infested section of town, we moved north 20 miles to Ridgefield, a tidy burg even today, even though the population has multiplied several times since 1963. I still go back there to see my best buddy, Tom Nash, and other friends, and to visit graves of those I knew, including Nana and a girl named Katie, who died young. She deserves her own book, written by me.

Later, my beloved cousin Bobby—tall, skinny and blond like me—was felled by leukemia at age 17 or 18. I was about 14 or so, and a mess. I was no longer reading a book a day and getting straight As with no effort. Puberty hit me like a shovel across the cranium, and when I awoke, dazed and confused, girls were the only thing on my mind, period! I was not one of those kids who could switch mental gears and do several tasks over the course of a day. Schoolwork was a waste of time, I thought, and so was any literature that did not educate me about how to get a girl naked. I read it all, good and perverted: Erich Fromm, de Sade, *My Secret Life* by "Walter," D. H. Lawrence, and scores of other books with sex as the central theme. This mindset underlies all of my thinking to this day, and I make no apologies. That's how I'm wired. I am a 74-inch pull-toy, a utility much like the little red wagon that contained my multi-colored toys when I was little. Nonetheless, John has educated, in his own way, the pull-toy quite thoroughly.

My cousin Bobby had the girl problem figured out. I had observed him closely, listening to every word he said as sexual gospel. He cracked wise, wore white T-shirts and drove a muscle car, and embodied the *American Graffiti* ethos. He had a different girlfriend every time I visited him in Franklin Square, Long Island. Those girls fawned over him with moist gazes, embodying a nubile look perfected by Natalie Wood. Oh what a scrumptious creature she was!

Bobby's grim prognosis was tearfully absorbed by the adults on my mother's side of the family. They went into a collective tailspin. The men went the philosophical and angry route. The women just could not bear the injustice and sadness and prematurity of the disease, for which there was no effective treatment. Nothing could so much as slow the strapping young man's decline. This was my initiation into viewing adults in a state of hopelessness, which can be scary for a teen who was coming to hate himself. I had learned my lesson well: Human beings were uniformly frail, temporary mammals motivated by love or fear, though this knowledge resided on a level that was largely inaccessible to my conscious mind.

Bobby's lovely older sister Carol Anne was engaged to be married. The wedding date was moved up so Bobby could attend. I vividly recall the scene as my parents prepared for the event. They hardly spoke at all. The church was packed. My uncle Bob, Bobby's dad, was a big wheel in the advertising business. Everything proceeded exactly like every other wedding I had attended until Bobby appeared at the church entrance. He was held up on either side by his high school peers. He looked to be six feet and 100 pounds, his face white as a sheet of paper. I was unnerved, as I had seen him in robust health only months previously. It was then that

I understood how adults held cancer in such awe and bleak foreboding. Perhaps as a defense mechanism, I developed a lifelong and active interest in the random nature of good and bad fortune, how luck plays such a decisive role in most everyone's life. Chaos became a close friend of mine.

Bobby passed on shortly afterwards and I went numb. I wasn't allowed to attend his funeral. It never occurred to my parents that I could have handled it well, as I had already been scarred for life by their blistering fights with threats of death in them. A close cousin's funeral was a one-time event that I understood occurred for us all, eventually. Then, with their provisional Lutheran beliefs, my parents stopped going to church. I was all for that, as the Jesus story was to me little more than an elaborate gambit promulgated by clever patriarchs, foremost among them Emperor Constantine, editor in chief of the Bible. I judged that the Jesus story would hold up only as long as it was the best afterlife fable in circulation. Subsequently, Muslims, Mormons, Scientologists, what have you, have adopted other patriarchal stories to cling to, and I am glad for them. Better for such people to feel they have a special role in the scheme of things than to have them moving about untethered to a belief system. As for Catholicism, I feel it was doomed the day somebody decided to replace the wooden cross symbol with a gold one, although that precious metal represents the church's goals quite well.

Without Bobby around to admire, I was left mostly alone to propel my family's green wooden rowboat on the shallow bass lake near my home. Sometimes my best friends Paul and Jonathan would fish with me. They were good guys and I miss them even today. I miss their dad, too. Francis Hines is a well-known artist who was my father's best friend at that time. I'd taught Bobby how to fish for bass one summer. It gave me a kick to teach him a manly skill while he regaled me with details about the girls in his life and how he won their affections. He was not a braggart, which gave credence to his role as a soft-peddling raconteur. I had learned that the world's activities hinged on stories, and on the natural treasures most girls guarded zealously.

The particulars of Bobby's escapades are lost on me now, no doubt obscured by the hormones that make a fool of me even today. At about age 15, in the first of a lifetime of social experiments both fair-minded and unseemly, I took a homely neighbor girl fishing, with the hope that she might touch me in return for the attention I was paying her. She squirmed at the sight of the worm on her hook, but that was about it. My thinly veiled entreaties fell on poorly sculpted ears and I was less than a gentleman when I docked the boat and shooed her home. As I watched her walk away, her curly black hair in a tight bun, it occurred to me that out on the lake she would have had few choices had I exerted myself like the beast I knew myself to be, as she was small and not a swimmer. Thus came the understanding of men's physical power over women and the essence of the term "gentleman," defined largely by the fact that men do not always heed their primal impulses.

Women would not be so tough on us if they could walk in our shoes for a day. Most men choose every day not to act on their true natures, and look how the culture responds—with exaltation of violence in the media, while healthy sex is denigrated as sinful. As some sort of corollary, I later developed a preference for women who understood the real nature of men and who had a constant awareness of the trouble men cause in the world. Such women bring gravitas to lovemaking, which I find ennobles the activity without taking the fun out of it.

I note here that I would not have presumed on the reader's time had I been the type of man who had at any point forced himself on a woman, or even struck a woman. I cannot tolerate that behavior at all. Even during the hazy 15-year stretch when I was drunk almost daily, I managed to swallow my anger along with the rivers of booze. However, I will add that, at low points in my life, I did engage in acts of emotional blackmail to achieve fornication, or copulation, depending on one's linguistic leanings. Women embody just about everything that brings me satisfaction, and I've learned to accept that fact about myself, although I admit to a deep wish that my artistic efforts gave me as much or more fulfillment. Alas, I would then be someone else, and I have worked way too hard to become who I am, someone I like and admire today.

As a teen, Holden Caulfield was a sniveler compared to me, a righteous miscreant at a young age, as I discovered alcohol at 16. Booze was the perfect antidote to the reality that there were no sex camps for young boys where a lad could mix with an endless array of insatiable nymphets (or so I would have it). Life was unfair and, for me, pimply and bug-eyed, booze not only took the edge off, it gave me a feeling of being removed and superior. It never occurred to me that booze was what was destroying my parents' relationship—and hence it could destroy me. Alcoholism is especially deadly in that it creates holes in one's awareness as it works its way into your life, like cancer. This accounted for some of the emotional blindness I suffered during those formative years. Such is the mindset of the compulsive, addictive personality.

Quietly descending into suburban teen madness, coveting every girl who paid me scant attention, I became something akin to a vampire. Female flesh was my preferred intoxicant but, failing in its pursuit, I always had booze to keep me going, numbing my feelings of rejection and worthlessness. There were some girls I was so enamored with I couldn't sleep from thinking about them, their prohibited warmth, their smiles, their giggles, the coy ways they found to say no. A half dozen or so of these girls I thought were perfect life partners at various points in my adolescence, yet I would not think of them in an erotic context for fear of there being no psychological exit from masturbatory daydreams. I had read enough Becket and Camus, and death had been on my mind for years. In my deep cynicism, love was never the point, as that special concept was for normal, stupid people to enjoy, those who did not comprehend the vastness of an indifferent universe in which love was merely a symptom of denial of one's ultimate meaninglessness. I was a very big-picture kind of guy, and girls didn't warm up to that. Go figure.

As I staggered through high school, convinced I would live the life of a cloistered, Nietzchean academic if the Russians didn't drop the bomb (I was certain they would), at 16 I fell hard for a blond classmate, a vivacious, smart, green-eyed beauty with a giggle that dismantled my isolationist worldview. Of course, she went out with older guys while warning me that I was drinking too much. I recall she lost her virginity to an *Up with People* type named Scooter or something like that. He wore tight white pants, I was told. He probably liked to listen to The Carpenters. Meanwhile, I was stunned into an alternative ecstasy by the first Led Zeppelin album. Still am in a trance from it on some level, as that record is a fine barometer of my adolescence. I already knew that America was made for the Scooters, not for cynics like me, but still, the inner torment persisted no matter how well I understood my alienation. As the flow of this type of information fueled my sense of being morbidly different, I accepted with a helpless nod the sinister nature of God, if there was one. My Scooter-loving friend wanted nothing from me but my humor, which I provided. Even today, women of a certain cast can cause me to feel like a lab rat stuck in a maze with no exit.

Such desire. It seems now that for weekends on end throughout the summer, I would fixate on the green-eyed blonde glistening on the local lakeside beach, each ripple of tanned muscle designed to inflame me. I generally do not go for blondes, but this girl's giggle was the animator of everything that mattered. The torturous feelings she caused put me in league with countless poets, suicides, madmen and motley curs down through the millennia. But the fact that I could commiserate with literary company did not help at all. Only cheap beer and wine kept me from the worst sort of self-destructive behavior, as there was no refuge at home, where my parents had at it over booze two or three nights a week. Forty years later, I still sleep with a pillow wrapped around my head, even though the noises coming through my window today are pleasant, seals and surf and squawking seabirds.

Thus, during my junior high and high school years, I was miserable, skin cracked and bleeding from rattled nerves and dehydration, horny all the time, all but uncaring about my appearance. Abandoning hope of an academic future, I guessed I would dissipate into an early grave. I recall a telling episode one day at a beach in Westport, Connecticut. I had gone there alone with no towel or sunscreen, just to think. When I came out of the water and lay down on the sand, I overheard a cute girl say to her friend about me: "Imagine hating yourself so much you don't even bring a towel to put under yourself." This was tough love from a stranger, and I heard it loud and clear. It's as if she said it yesterday. It was true; I hated myself then, with my gawky body, terrible skin problems, and a sense that I was put on earth to contemplate my own purposelessness. Booze kept the feelings repressed.

In 1969, the summer of my 16th year, I found the long-sought goal in the arms of a buddy's 20-year-old sister at a party in Greenwich, where my father was still a junior high school principal when he wasn't acting and singing in *The Fantasticks, Born Yesterday* or Gilbert and Sullivan extravaganzas. The sex was brief and meaningless. I couldn't look the girl in the eye. But once that initial encounter was behind me, I came to agree that all the fuss about sex was warranted. Everywhere I looked, I saw sex as a motive. So was the avoidance of sex, or the fear of sex, or the masking of motives related to sex, and on and on. Still an eager reader, I viewed all art from a hormone-saturated perspective and, for some reason, I thought I was the only one doing so, as most guys my age were smiling and laughing and playing sports. We humans are most naïve when we proclaim our own uniqueness or even specialness, yet undeterred, I foraged among the younger girls of the quality western Connecticut towns, seeking to bed as many as possible, convinced that this was what Mother Nature intended. The fact that girls had feelings was merely one of the obstacles to be overcome.

The first serious symptom of my overall spiritual sickness was a bleeding ulcer at 17, which put me in the hospital. The only adult who took useful notice was my social studies teacher and counselor Dirk Bollenback, who took me aside and asked me what was wrong. I wouldn't betray my parents, so I assured him nothing was wrong at home. My condition did not stop my pals from smuggling beer into my hospital room. The various shrinks I saw took me for an alien. They just could not figure me out. I would say that I was very angry at any God that had put me there. I hated that I had the ability to consider man's hapless fate, knowing that God would kill me off with no hope for answers to the big questions that He had posed. It is the most vicious of conundrums, and yes, dear readers, I knew then that love was the answer. I just didn't know how to find it, or realize that I was too sick then to attract a healthy partner. All the while, the blues-driven dirges of heavy metal groups animated my soul as it sought a way toward the light. It would be more than a decade down the tunnel of my 20s before that light appeared.

Hostile existentialism was a mode that worked for me in some cases, as some of my sister's friends found me amusing enough to disrobe and then some. I was grateful, but not for long. My ego demanded I bed not those girls whom I viewed as similarly disenfranchised, but the more visible girls, the icons, if not the exalted cheerleaders themselves. I was into humping female symbols of the establishment. Girls wearing Ridgefield High School orange and black Tigers' socks and nothing else would have increased my ardor. That wish for the over-achieving, ruddy faced, Ivy-league bound group went mostly unrequited. At lunchtime in high school, I could be found outside on the swings, swigging white wine wrapped in a brown paper bag, or driving aimlessly all over town with a mild beer buzz.

Along the way I discovered porn in lurid forms, including the aforementioned *My Secret Life,* by "Walter," a Victorian nobleman who plowed willing damsels in 19th-century Europe. Films in New York's Times Square were worth a train trip, including one titled *Stalag 69,* a revolting, violent piece of fascist trash porn that skewered whatever innocence I had left. On the plus side, my favorite film of all time, *Five Easy Pieces,* was released in 1970. It was nothing less than revelatory for me. The character played by Jack Nicholson embodied my mindset perfectly. I have watched that film perhaps 50 times over the years.

High school moroseness was broken by a few events that shook me to the core. The prettiest girl in the school, as breathtaking as an 18-year-old girl can be, was killed when her Corvair slid off a road in a light rain. To this day she remains the most gorgeous girl I have ever seen, sort of a cross between Jane Fonda in *Cat Ballou* and Brigitte Bardot in her prime. Just an absurd specimen whose number came up. Also, the football team's star quarterback was stricken with leukemia. He died as quickly as Bobby had passed. The entire school population became unglued by both events. When I visit the graves of those I knew in Ridgefield, his gray stone serves as a particularly poignant sentinel, like the monolith in another of my favorite films, *2001: A Space Odyssey,* emblematic of the dreams of youth, dashed to nothingness by cancer. This young athlete was a great person, one of the few jocks I respected. Once again, I had crossed paths with the Big C and it had made a permanent impression.

Also in 1970, the film *Love Story* opened, starring the delicious Ali MacGraw, just my type. Our high school organized a bus trip to see it. I chose instead to get into my 1960 Chevy Brookwood station wagon and get drunk with some buddies. That big wagon had a Blue Flame inline six cylinder motor and three-speed manual transmission on the steering column. I put a ratty mattress in the back and two Styrofoam coolers, one for beer, one for wine. Oh, the girls heard plenty of lies in that rolling den of iniquity! The huge Chevy eventually gave way to a tiny black VW, which curbed my enthusiasm for sex on wheels.

For a week, the girls walked around teary-eyed, recalling scenes from *Love Story,* whose tagline was "Love means never having to say you're sorry." Oh, really? I did eventually see the movie, at the green-eyed blonde's urging, and was I ever sorry. I thought it was perhaps the worst film of all time and my opinion has not changed since then, although *The English Patient* gives it some competition. More recently, the sexual-identity debacle *Boys Don't Cry,* about a female common thief who wants to be a boy, was another paradigm of Hollywood crap. These dishonest films are manipulative to a profane degree.

What kind of example does *Love Story* set for kids trying to deal with grief in the real world? Death from disease is not always something we learn from; I'd figured that out early on. Ask the ghosts of the many millions of people who have died not knowing one healthy, contented day on earth. To look death in the eye and remain stoic is admirable, but our culture should not require stoicism as the mark of courage. It should be equally fine to break down and scream at the moon until one is hoarse. One might go gently into that good night, but why add guilt to the minds of those who cannot muster courage in their final moments? My cousin Bobby looked honestly lost and defeated on his sister's wedding day, and I do not think less of him for that. Any emotion earned honestly should be respected.

Hazily, I recall that the last day I attended high school was in April of my senior year. Most weekends, I had been taking the train to the Fillmore East concert arena in New York City, to be enthralled by Led Zeppelin, Jethro Tull, Jeff Beck, Spirit, Janis Joplin with Big Brother and the Holding Company, and various other acts that have stood the test of time. In New York's East Village, I tried marijuana and hated it. But I also tried older, nihilistic girls who were sexually selfish. I loved them. They were so content to lie back and let me work them over. Whether I climaxed or not, they didn't care. Their aloofness was fantastic. Thus grew my number one desire: to satisfy my partners. More on this later. One of my former heroes, Woody Allen, put this concept in perfect context in a scene from *Play It Again, Sam.* A cute, urbane girl is in an otherwise empty museum gallery, gazing at a painting. Woody's character looks her up and down and asks her what she's doing Saturday night. She says she's committing suicide. After the briefest pause, he asks her "What about Friday night?" That was me, looking for opportunities for sensory pleasure before the shroud of death enveloped us all.

I graduated from high school in order to remove my dark presence from the school system, and also because my ACT score was close to perfect, despite the fact that I had failed English in my junior year. Adrift, I worked for a year at a local bookstore and drove a big truck to pick up discounted books by the half ton. One evening, returning with a load of books (the metaphor is not lost on me), I stopped at a diner and picked up a hooker. I found her purposeful and efficient, but the experience left me more hollow than before, so I was not a repeat customer.

Next up was a trip to Europe for a couple of months, stopping in London before heading off to Denmark and Sweden, the homes of my forebears. London was the urban embodiment of my personality, and for decades it was my favorite city, though San Francisco is my choice today. My first weekend in London, I had an encounter with an American girl who said, as she was leaving my hotel room, "I wish I could stay forever," a line for which I had no retort at the time. Oh, was she hot! I stood in the hotel hallway in my underwear, clutching a bottle of scotch as she wandered tearfully away.

A few days later I found the underside of that storied city and my situation improved. I was robbed of 20 pounds, but the thief turned out to be a porcelain-skinned bohemian chick who slept with me for two nights, so I called it even. This was the weekend Stanley Kubrick's *A Clockwork Orange* opened, so the subject of crime was in the air. A few days after that I lucked upon two drug-addled sisters. In return for a warm place to sleep and some hot meals, they allowed me to take them by turns, and they wore me out. I became convinced that an erect penis could divide any problem into manageable component parts.

After that I sailed to Denmark to see my paternal grandmother and then to Sweden, where the girls were relaxed, curious about America, and accommodating. On reflection, I'm surprised I ever returned to the States, although I probably would have drunk myself to death in Scandinavia, as is a time-honored custom. So many kindred spirits adrift on a metaphorical iceberg of self-annihilation. What's not to like?

Back stateside, I played the enamored imbecile, hitchhiking to the green-eyed blonde's college only to be rejected yet again. She had a poster of a donkey on the wall in her dorm that said "Good Ass Is Hard to Find." Only recently I threw out all her letters to me from that horrible time. It only took my heart 40 years to catch up with what my mind knew well even back then.

I was expected to attend college, so I chased a girl to a big university in the Southwest and stayed for a year. I hated everything about that school except for the one Native American girl who typed my papers at 100 wpm as I dictated them to her. I returned to Connecticut, mostly to keep my father from killing my family, which he threatened to do all the time whenever I was on the phone with him. By this point the reader no doubt has the picture of a self-destructive guy with no future. I mean me, not my father, though the appraisal could apply equally to either or both of us.

I got a job as a jack-of-all-trades at my local newspaper. My alcoholism had been in full sway for nearly 10 years by the time I was in my mid-20s, and my ambition was measured in hours, making it through the day until I could get loaded in the late afternoon at the bars in town where I had revolving credit. My sex life was intermittent at best. I would pick up a drunk of the other gender and it would last all of two hours, maybe four. Names and details were not important. A real girlfriend was out of the question. One letter I received from an exquisite beauty named Cindy, who liked my Humphrey Bogart impression, read "Get lost. Need I say more?" I deserved a worse send-off, as my drinking took me down and down. Some of the things I did behind the wheel of a car and some of the things I said to people haunt me to this day. I have a great deal of remorse for all of it. We drunks don't get up in the morning—or the afternoon, for that matter—with a plan to create mayhem in others' lives. In my late 20s, when I lived in Manhattan, I might start my afternoon at the Plaza Hotel drinking with Salvador Dali and conclude the bender at 2 A.M. in the Bowery or in Harlem, playing pool for dollar drafts with individuals of less artistic accomplishment. Often I was the only white guy in the Royal Flush Bar, way uptown. Somehow I managed to find the D train and make it home.

Similarly, in my early and mid-20s back in Connecticut, on a typical night, the descent would commence in swank New Canaan, where my buddies and I would approach Ivy League girls with the announcement that we were on moisture patrol and that the salami needed hiding. My favorite line was "We'll go to your place, I'll put it in halfway, and if you don't like it, I'll take it out." Then I would backpeddle, deflect the target's anger, and be clever in a self-mocking way. Tough going, that route. Some of my handsomer buddies got action with that abusive style, but not me, except for one time when I cajoled a tearful brunette out to my car. She did what I wanted but slapped my face, too. More often I concluded an evening in a bowling alley parking lot in blue-collar Brewster, New York, receiving oral dispensations in my car from poorly nourished girls with self-esteem lower than mine. These nocturnal endeavors seemed just desserts at the time, for both parties.

A high point would be a week or two each summer on Nantucket, where my luck was better, perhaps because the hotly bookish girls from Boston took so much pride in their jaded attitude toward sex. "We're all going to die anyway, so why do I shave my legs again? Over here, schmuck; take it if you want it." Perfect!

Without taking anything away from the marvelous women in my personal history, especially those with whom I have enjoyed long-term relationships, there has been only one woman in my intimate history who knew me intuitively. Little needed to be said. This was in the late '70s, when I was truly a mess. My beloved Yankees were on top in the American League and I was on top of a few dim-bulb narcissists. Then along came an older woman in a bad marriage. Somehow she knew just when I needed a whisper of encouragement, a frenzy of vengeful copulation, caring admonishment, or the slow administration of oral favors given or received. She was highly educated, a delightful dinner companion, decked out in Italian designer clothes, yet she would purposely raise her white tennis skirt for me when I pinned her against a tree on a golf course. I certainly accept my role in the everyday give and take, in the negotiations between the sexes, but it is cathartic for me to relate the brief time I spent in fleeting harmony with that fine woman. When I was too drunk to perform sexually, she would play lewd games in front of me so as to rile my id for later. How she avoided adopting the usual inhibitions of most American women is a mystery to me. Such wild creatures are unbearably rare.

With her, I never had to jump through the hoops of discussion and reassurance that one usually needs to clear to establish a balanced bond where both parties benefit, making the sum of the two persons greater than the whole. Creating that third, greater entity can be so rewarding, yet it is often a very fragile thing. The requirement to talk things through to keep resentments from building is at the core of most good relationships. In fact, the most common way men signal that they want out of a union is to clam up. This mode does not apply to me, however, as I can be all but silent in a relationship and still be quite content. Perhaps I am essentially a solitary being, although I crave company from time to time. Conversely, when I lived alone, I would shrink a bit emotionally. I just don't know the answer.

In the early '80s, I came back to New York City and moved in with Paula, who would become my wife. I had known her since childhood, when she was my sister's best friend. She too had endured the abusive ravings of an alcoholic father. Mostly due to her efforts, and with help from her terrific mother, we bought a great little top-floor one-bedroom co-op on tree-lined Bedford Street in the West Village. She got me a job at the men's clothing designer firm she worked for and we somehow put a life together, despite my active alcoholism and the emotional distance it created. We shared many, many good times and, in a deeply abiding way that will inspire me forever, Paula taught me how to love and to begin to love myself. What can a man say about a woman that special, who put up with crazy alcoholic behavior and then nurtured me during the shaky early years of sobriety? What a marvelous person she is. Still, many of those last nights of blackout drinking were tough on her. I would disappear into gambling dens and other black holes, where I fostered odd acquaintanceships with an assortment of shady characters. One night a guy paid me $500 cash to drive a car to Newark, New Jersey. Now you know as much about that gig as I do.

On December 6, 1984, I awoke to yet another in a string of brutal hangovers. In recent weeks I had been getting my mail delivered to Chumley's Bar across the street, partly for the mailman's amusement and also because I thought it better to scan and discard overdue bills in the near darkness of a pub than in the accusing glare of home. But something broke in me that December morning. I had had enough. An inner voice said "You must decide today—live or die." I chose a 30-day rehab program and have not had a drop of booze since, nor any unprescribed mood-changing drug. That doesn't mean things went well thereafter. My life got worse for a year after I gave up booze and the cocaine that kept me awake enough to drink.

Thus, 1985 was my worst year ever in psychic terms, as I was petrified to try to learn how to live without my chosen general anesthetics. Paranoid and sensitive to every slight, I was a 32-year-old guy who could barely make it to the corner to buy milk and bread, let alone work gainfully, or be there to support a partner. I would consider killing myself because my soon-to-be wife, a magna-cum-laude graduate from Smith College, had beaten me at a few games of Scrabble. But I was clean and determined not to fall back into my old habits. Yet the night terrors almost did me in, as my mind healed in ways that were gothic in their horror. For a few months, I was scared to sleep. One morning the images got so bad I awoke sweating at 4 A.M., slipped on a coat, and headed down to the subway, intending to step in front of a #1 train. I waited on the Christopher Street platform for 20 minutes or so before I got bored, gave up on the idea, went home and slid back into bed. Paula was unaware of my foray. Impatience has saved me more than once. Someone has written that patience is the mildest form of despair. I wish I had time to think about that.

Inevitably, I tried to work. After tragicomic stints of temping at law firms and in telemarketing, my late and dear friend Nick Deane, who was a publishing executive, gave me freelance writing work. I commenced a long career as a business journalist. My self-esteem rose and my thoughts became more focused and, more importantly, well-structured. I could again match tops with the pots they fit. I saw a great therapist, T. J. Elliott, who informed me that "Everyone is doing the best they can, all the time," and "Action is character." I learned that I was a garden-variety drunk who relied on a kind of postmodern priapism for a meager identity and that it was time to grow up. I thought I took this direction pretty well, but it turns out I was fooling myself.

Despite my intentions to the contrary, I was still incapable of true intimacy, which I understand today stemmed from an inability to allow another person to know me completely. I engaged in superficial sex without engaging my spirit, for I surely felt I could not survive a truly intimate experience, nor could I ever trust the person who might have held that knowledge of me. These are all symptoms of self-pity, the downfall of most people who give up on themselves. Today, I am in a place 180 degrees from that emotional turmoil: I fear *not* being known intimately as much as I once feared being known. True, some of this progress is borne on the advance of years, but it has more to do with the personal work I've done to better myself, and this includes sexual relationships. My primary need to satisfy my partner has given me a sense of usefulness that has proved indispensable as a psychological foundation. Sure, I enjoy being sexually stimulated as much as the next man, but the boundless curiosity I have about female sexual response always leads the way.

As I sobered up, I found that underlying chronic depression and anxiety were dominating feelings I could neither accept nor manage well, and I withdrew from my wife. I didn't know then that I was not qualified to be anyone's life partner, much less the partner of a woman as fine as Paula. In time, I came to heed the siren call of Los Angeles. Trapped by a psychic condition I have yet to understand fully, I ended my marriage in 1996 and moved to L.A., where I had a rough time of it. In my 40s, I was living alone for the first time. There were several relationships, ranging from an hour to several weeks, but I was, as they say, unavailable emotionally. One relationship was important, with a sweet redhead who needed rehab herself. I treasure her friendship still, as she is the most courageous person I know, persevering with a good attitude in the face of numerous medical and emotional problems. The Hollywood girls were fun, mostly, but crazy enough to set me somewhat straight about casual sex. Many of them had been traumatized in their youth, which led me on wild expeditions through their minds to get them to climax. Sometimes I found the way, sometimes not.

Back in New York, I had worked with a woman named Debbie. She was sweet as could be and had a young daughter, Jillian, from a previous marriage. Debbie and I commenced dating long distance. She has an almost mystical way of getting me to open up, the way good women do when they love somebody and are intent on getting the best of that person to emerge. I learned to talk about my feelings and became active in Alcoholics Anonymous. Jillian and I became buddies and, as a trio, we began to look like a ready-made family. But there were considerable hurdles to be cleared, including Jillian's wish to finish high school in New York and my uncertain career as a freelance writer.

But by the late '90s, I was churning out articles for umpteen business journals and making a decent living riding the Internet and the NASDAQ waves. Then one summer day in 1999, I noticed that my urination stream was a little different than it had been all my adult life. Breaking a long pattern of avoiding doctors, off I went to a walk-in clinic, where I was seen by a Dr. Kevorkian, no relation to the plug-puller. She commenced saving my life with a simple blood test, the PSA.

Two

DIAGNOSIS

I'm a huge fan of science, and have no superstitions or irrational fears. Thus, if science tells me a disease can spread rapidly without generating any clear symptoms, I'm not going to dismiss such assertions as over-protective or as part of a scam perpetrated by the big drug companies. Still, in the case of my prostate cancer, I was lucky to have it discovered at an early stage. Virtually all the literature recommends one begin testing at age 50, and for months following my surgery I lobbied the American Cancer Society to change their recommendation to age 45. One can imagine the added costs to HMOs if such a recommendation were instituted, so of course I got nowhere. Thus, men who get prostate cancer in their 40s had better be lucky if they are going to catch it in time. Moreover, the younger one is, the more aggressive the cancer is, generally speaking. It comes down to personal initiative or good advice from a trusted source. Knowing that thousands of men in their 40s will die from prostate cancer anyway does not make this effort to inform any easier to write, that I can tell you. And then there are the many thousands of men who will simply not go to the doctor for regular check-ups. Such men are easy prey to the silent killer prostate cancer. Is that you or your friend of 30 years? Does it run in your family? Life-saving answers may be a blood test away.

Fully 15 percent of men in America will have prostate cancer in their lifetimes, most in their 60s and older, but thanks to improving diagnostic methods and treatment, most of those so afflicted will be diagnosed in an early phase of the disease, when there are several treatment options available. Sadly, tens of thousands of American men die of the disease each year, and many more worldwide. Nearly all of them could be saved by heightened awareness, overcoming fear of the unknown, and taking action.

Not every man with prostate cancer would so claim, but there was a silver lining in my case. My ordeal put the gifts in my life into sharp focus; interesting people, exciting ideas and fruitful experiences are the rule in my life today, not the exception. I am very grateful, as it has been 10 years since my cancerous prostate was removed. Over this last decade, I have learned a great deal about not just the recovery process, but also about the pitfalls men face prior to diagnosis, and after diagnosis but prior to surgery. In the United States alone, many thousands of men have prostate cancer right now yet do not know it. Unchecked, this malignancy may grow beyond the prostate gland capsule, metastasizing to other parts of the body before any symptoms are felt. By then it is too late to cure it.

So who are you guys who are either afraid to go to the doctor or afraid to proceed with treatment? How many of you think you have no time to go to the doctor? How many of you feel you are taking care of yourself, so you must be in good health? Would you rather take a day off to find out you have early prostate cancer and live to be 80, or continue on the way you are and be cut down at 60? The fact is, a man could be a top senior class marathoner and be fatally afflicted with prostate cancer that has yet to metastasize to a place in his body where it causes pain. It took me five years to get one of my auto mechanics to heed my advice about seeing a urologist, even though he had abnormal urination in his 40s. Turns out he has BPH (benign prostatic hyperplasia, a relatively harmless though annoying enlargement of the gland), but it could have gone another way. If prostate cancer runs in your family, and you are 40 or older, you should be getting tested annually, period. The disease has a very strong genetic component, almost to the point of a guarantee that a son will get it if his father has had it. The question then becomes: At what age? My brother Steve, who's 50 as I write this, may get prostate cancer, but I hope he's 85 at the time, if indeed he is dealt that card. My father's brother John had prostate surgery in his early 70s and lived into his middle 80s, so the malformed gene certainly has made its presence known on the paternal side of my extended family. Of those men diagnosed in an early phase, many will choose a radical prostatectomy as primary treatment, with the hope that all, or nearly all, of the cancer will be removed with the excision of the gland. Not to belabor the point, but with years to reflect on the matter, I would choose this option again, given what I know today.

It should be obvious that the people I most want to reach are those men who shy away from physical exams and from surgery. Their partners may share in the responsibility of getting their men to a doctor for regular check-ups. I know plenty of otherwise intelligent, highly functional men age 50 and up who go to the doctor only when they feel something is wrong. I cannot stress this strongly enough: Shirking doctors is potentially deadly behavior. Specifically, a simple blood test called a PSA (prostate specific antigen) test can usually reveal whether or not the prostate gland is normal. A digital rectal exam (DRE) is another detection procedure. That's when a urologist places a gloved, lubed finger in a man's rectum to feel if the shape of the prostate gland has been distorted by cancer. A DRE takes a few seconds, and if you find that prospect uncomfortable, I suggest you weigh some of the alternatives.

Some men are more prone to the disease than others. For some reason unknown to science, African-American men are more predisposed to early prostate cancer, so if you are of that race, you should get a PSA every year commencing at age 40. PSA testing becomes critical to maintaining health, so make it a yearly routine. To repeat, if there is any prostate cancer in your family history, testing should commence at age 40 regardless of ethnic background. Men owe it to themselves and to their loved ones to get this painless, noninvasive test every year. It prolonged my life, perhaps by decades.

Deadly thinking is perhaps best exemplified by a friend of a friend of mine, a tough 50-something professional whose PSA numbers were worse than mine were when I had two tumors growing in my prostate. This tough guy acknowledged that there might be something wrong with him, but he would not consider treatment until he felt symptoms. There was no changing his mind. So for two years he waited for a medical epiphany, until one day he noticed some trouble urinating and, worse, back pain. In such cases, the back pain may be caused by prostate cancer that has spread from the prostate gland to the seminal vesicles, then to nearby lymph nodes and then to the pelvis and spine. By that point, not only is it too late to cure the cancer, but the prognosis for any treatment is bleak, and survival time from diagnosis is almost always brief, perhaps a year or two. This guy disappeared from my friend's life to parts unknown, perhaps to where elephants go.

By contrast, if prostate cancer is caught when it is confined to the gland, the prognosis is usually very good to excellent. This scenario was typified by my case. I stress the sexual elements of my story because there is not much explicit material available about sex after prostate cancer treatment. This probably stems from the simple fact that, in a Judeo-Christian culture, discussions of sex are still taboo for many people. I find this attitude oppressive, so in some respects this book is also a rebuke to an immature norm that needs to be replaced by a healthy openness toward one of life's greatest joys. There are no such hang-ups in Europe or most of Asia, for example.

While I do not seek to offend people, this is a book for adults. There is no gratuitous sexual content in this book, but much of what I experienced in recovery requires graphic description to properly make a point, either about prostate cancer or human sexuality. I trust readers will appreciate this approach. Clearly, the profile of prostate cancer has been raised in recent years, but coverage of the sexual aftereffects of treatment lags well behind coverage of other aspects of treatment and recovery.

Certainly, not every man with prostate cancer chooses surgery. There are radiation treatments and hormone therapies. Men who have gone those routes should tell their stories, and there is a plethora of doctors' opinions and medical literature concerning those approaches. On the treatment horizon, gene therapy holds considerable promise and perhaps someday soon doctors will tailor treatments to each man's genetic make-up. Genes could be used to diminish tumor development, or such research may lead to vaccine-type preventatives. But in my case, I found the idea of cutting the disease out of me to be the most appealing of the several daunting alternatives. Which brings me back to Doctor Kevorkian.

At the risk of sounding like a down and out detective, by 1999 I was divorced and living in Hollywood, working out of a 1920s vintage apartment just down the hill from the famous Hollywood sign. I had finished working one warm afternoon and decided to go through some old papers. This led to pondering unfinished business, which prompted the realization that I had not had a physical exam in some time, a couple of years at least. Plus, I had noticed a mildly altered urine stream, not a problem per se, but an annoyance. At times there was a spray, rather than a stream. There was not a hint of pain.

There was a utilitarian walk-in clinic near my apartment, which somehow suited my mood at the time. As I signed in and waited my turn to see the solo practitioner who ran the place, I was about 15 pounds overweight on a six-foot two-inch frame and feeling pretty good all around. I figured the doctor would tell me to exercise more, eat better and send me packing.

My turn came and I went in to see Dr. Kevorkian, not Dr. Doom of course, but a likable, slender woman with the mellifluous first name Siranoush. She gave me the once over, asked a few questions and had a nurse take some blood. Noting my age, 46, on the intake form she said "you'll be 50 soon enough so why don't we throw in a PSA test while we're at it?"

I had no idea what a PSA test was, perhaps a Pakistani airline work application, I joked at the time, but there was seriousness in her tone as she explained it. I went ahead with it, despite the added $70 lab fee. Many readers will know that a PSA is a simple test that measures trace amounts of a prostate specific antigen, which is a protein in the blood. The key fact is that this protein is indeed specific to the prostate and to no other body part. Four nanograms (4.0 in typical numerical parlance) per milliliter or less is considered in the normal range for this antigen. Basically, the lower the number, the better. For example, my tests today come back <0.1.

A few busy days went by. I had all but forgotten about the doctor visit. Then the phone rang early one morning, with one of the clinic's administrators on the line. The doctor wanted to see me, she said, to discuss the results of the PSA test. I asked if the doctor could speak with me over the phone, but she wasn't having it. With a metallic taste in my mouth, I jumped in my car and drove to the clinic. During the 15-minute ride, I contemplated the strong possibility that I had cancer. Self-pity kicked in as I conjured images of my long-dead cousin. Would I soon begin wasting away, well before I had achieved a modest level of happiness? Had God perhaps snapped out of His splendid indifference to issue me a reprieve for my alcoholism? Was He now cashing in my chips because I had displayed insufficient gratitude for my second chance? Such were the remnants of the insidious religious training of my youth. About halfway to the clinic I became very, very sad and pulled into a 7-Eleven. I bought a soda and sat on a concrete ledge to compose myself. A homeless guy gave me a dollar. Just kidding. Old joke, couldn't resist. I called Denis, an old friend from rehab back in New York, on a payphone, but he wasn't home. I didn't leave a message.

The clinic was empty when I got there, so Dr. Kevorkian saw me right away. With an unreadable expression on her face, she said that my PSA was elevated, at about 8, which put me in a very gray area, the range for either cancer or perhaps only BPH. She suggested I see a urologist, with the qualified warning that if I did have cancer, it was probably in an early stage and could likely be cured. I remember mumbling questions about how that could be done, and I recall only a few words from her answer: surgery, radiation, hormone therapy. Little of what she said was comforting, so as I drove home and I kept the word "cured" foremost in my mind. I began to gird for a protracted medical and financial ordeal, as I was uninsured. My cousin Bobby, I knew, never heard the word "cured" in his final days.

Once home, I fired up my PC and logged onto the Internet, where I knew there would be plenty of information available on cancer of the prostate. Sure enough, within hours I had a working knowledge of the disease, although there were many disturbing aspects that went beyond the obvious death-dealing one. At first, I focused on details related to my personal PSA score.

From what I was learning, with a PSA in the single digits, it was likely that if I had cancer, it was confined to the prostate gland and thus could be cured most definitively by surgery. This idea was simple and appealing: cut out the offending part and that should be that. Radiation scared me more than surgery, as I had seen how incredibly sick one could become from such treatments. In the early 1990s, a friend, Tom, the bravest man I know, had beaten lung cancer against very daunting odds. He endured brutal radiation therapy over a long period, yet never wavered in his resolve and good humor. Another dear friend of mine, Nick, mentioned earlier, has recently died of lung cancer. I can thank the tobacco industry and our greedy governments for sharing the blame in both cases. On the face of it, how can it be that selling tobacco is still legal with all we know about its effects? Imagine trying to get it legalized today, if tobacco were a newly discovered plant? It would have no chance in hell of getting to consumer shelves, and yet it remains a multi-billion dollar industry that does no one anything but harm. Amazing world we live in, isn't it?

On the scientific front, in recent years, analysis of the PSA test has skewed more towards the rate of change of the reading, rather than just the number. PSA velocity is now accepted as an important measurement in and of itself. Thus, even if one's PSA is under 4.0, if it has changed, say, from 1.0 to 3.0 in a year, that bump in the number would be enough for some urologists to recommend a biopsy. You can bet this will set off another round of hostility in the boardrooms of insurers and HMOs, as the doctors seek to test vulnerable subjects and the paper-pushers seek to keep costs down.

Perhaps advances on the use of PSA are forthcoming. In 2007, a new prostate cancer test was announced, which measures a blood protein called EPCA-2. This test was found to be 94 percent accurate, a much better result than the standard PSA blood test. The PSA has a high incidence of registering false positives and catches only 85 percent of prostate cancers, although it caught mine, of course. This new test should help reduce the number of men who get prostate biopsies, since every year, out of 1.6 million men in the United States who suffer the intrusive hollow biopsy needle, only 200,000 are found to have cancer. Moreover, the new test helps determine if the cancer has spread beyond the prostate capsule, which in itself is hugely significant. Although the new test still faces FDA hurdles, the public should be benefiting from it soon. Further down the diagnostic road, look for a urine-based test that should scare no one. There's no reason, other than fear and ignorance, why tens of thousands of American men have to die each year from prostate cancer.

As for prostate cancer's causes, a genetic predisposition appears to be the only specific indicator, yet I have willingly participated in several medical surveys since my ordeal, as institutions explore its causes. I predict that a cure lies in our DNA and in the resultant inoculations that will eventually be made from it. Call it a sculpted bullet theory. In retrospect, the decision to get the PSA test at the walk-in clinic is one of the more hair-raising aspects of my story. I made the decision to get tested based on a very weak hunch that it was best to be thorough. Dr. Kevorkian mentioned the PSA test offhandedly, and would not have pushed me if I had displayed any resistance. She probably knew that only a small fraction of cases of prostate cancer are found in white men age 46 and under. If I had followed the American Cancer Society's recommendation, I'd have been a dead man walking. The cancer would have had three and a half more years to grow undetected prior to my 50th birthday. Then there would have been the matter of motivating myself to get to a doctor's office.

The evening I got the results, I discussed the news with Debbie, who is exceptionally level-headed when it comes to medical matters. She reminded me that it was only one test and that I should get another one to confirm the initial results. This struck me as inarguable advice, and the next day I set about finding a urologist, not a straightforward proposition as I did not know anyone who had urinary or related problems. My memory of the search process is foggy, as I was in a zombified state, but I recall wandering randomly into a doctor's office in a Hollywood hospital known for processing a lot of distressed people off the street, like me. As I sat in a dingy waiting room, a somewhat wild-eyed, unkempt urologist stormed out to speak gruffly to a patient. I quickly rose and exited. There was no way I was entrusting my body, my private parts, or anything else to that guy. He could have gotten a role as one of the villagers in the film *Borat*.

Always a danger in the kitchen, I went out to a fast food place to try to choke a meal down. I was upset and must have looked awful. Another homeless guy—never mind. I went grocery shopping and went home, in despair but nonetheless very grateful to Dr. Kevorkian for her thoroughness. A couple of months after my surgery, I would stop by the clinic and bring her flowers. She was shocked, reporting that I was the only patient she'd ever had who made such a gesture. It seemed the least I should do. Next time I'll give her a copy of this book, as she's responsible for setting it in motion.

Once again, I went to Debbie for a suggestion. She had needed a doctor the last time she'd visited me in L.A. and had been referred to Dr. Ronald Sue, a fine internist who practiced in a private, well-ordered facility on L.A.'s west side. Debbie had been very impressed by Dr. Sue's professionalism, and suggested that I get a recommendation from him. I called him and, without hesitation, he said: "Call Fred Kuyt. He works in the building. He'll take good care of you." I never thanked Dr. Sue properly, as Fred has taken extraordinarily good care of me over the ensuing years. Plus, I gained a friend, always a good thing. Debbie, however, did stop in to thank Dr. Sue while I was in the hospital. She does things like that, paragon of civilization that she is.

Fred Kuyt is a great guy and a very careful doctor. Even though he has been through his share of personal trials, he is a happy person, gifted and circumspect. I all but required a happy doctor to offset my inconsistent, depression-prone mindset. Many readers will identify with the process of recovering on an unsure emotional foundation. The process of diagnosis, surgery and recovery forced me to take a very deep look inside myself, to tap into resources I had no idea existed. It was very humbling to learn that my self-knowledge was so incomplete. Gaining more of this hard-won knowledge has been one of the most valuable byproducts of this experience. Know thyself and life becomes less difficult.

For readers facing surgery, radiation or other cancer-related procedures, I cannot stress how important it is to find a urologist who is not just a good physician and surgeon, but a good communicator as well. He or she should be an effective counselor, with the strong verbal skills to explain the details of all the changes you will experience. Once the shock of the diagnosis wears off, your ears will become radar dishes tuned to your doctor's words. In contrast to my experience with Fred, I've received e-mails from men from around the world in the wake of the *Washington Post* article, telling me that their surgeons told them nothing beyond the nuts-and-bolts basics, pun intended. These doctors are glorified plumbers, though I suspect they are paid about the same. The elementary counseling they offer is on the order of "You'll be in the hospital for three to five days, you'll wear a catheter for a few weeks and then, with time, you'll probably be fine." This attitude curdles my blood. I believe that rather than take on the risk, responsibility, and effort of fully disclosing the ramifications of the various treatment regimens, many well-meaning doctors play on our culture's mandate that men should tough it out. These doctors meet their minimum obligations and get the job done, but I sense that it is too often up to patients to ask crucial questions. And many patients, befuddled by trepidation and ignorant of complications that may arise, do not even know which questions to ask.

Fred administered my first DRE. For once I managed to refrain from making jokes about how he should have first treated me to dinner and a show. That painless probing proved inconclusive, which is not unusual, as almost half of prostate cancers are not detectable by a DRE. A lab assistant took blood for a PSA and I went home feeling confident in Fred's abilities, but guardedly wary about my overall medical situation.

Two days later the results were in, and my PSA had scored 7+, similar to the number registered at the clinic. Fred then had me get a third measurement, instructing me to not ejaculate for at least 48 hours prior to the test. Sexual activity can elevate PSA levels, so I followed his instructions and scored 6.2. Better, but still abnormal. Fred insisted I have a biopsy of the prostate gland.

In a few days I made my way to the office of one of Fred's colleagues, a pleasant individual who was matter of fact about his very specific job. In a TRUS (transrectal ultrasound) biopsy, the specialist's hand is guided by video images created by ultrasound. A plastic probe the width of a pinky finger is lubricated and inserted into the rectum. Then, a spring-loaded needle snaps forward to harpoon the fleshy wall between the rectum and the prostate gland, which abuts the other side of the wall. The lightning quick punctures of the prostate gland do not hurt per se, but they do make you wince. One is excused for feeling very vulnerable during and after the procedure. To say it felt strange would be understating the matter considerably.

The needle is hollow and extracts tissue from both the innermost and outer parts of the gland. In my case, there were six probes (called a sextant biopsy), which provided a representative sampling of the walnut-sized prostate. Other doctors might take 8 or 10 samples, or currently, two dozen. Five minutes and $1,200 later, the doctor was peeling off his gloves. It took awhile to clean myself of the applied lubricant and I was grateful that the pretty nurses did not smirk as I squishily meandered out of the office. The samples were sent to a pathology lab. (Note: Try to find the word "squishily" anywhere else in adult literature. For fellow word freaks out there, the term to describe a word used only once in recorded literature is "hapaxlegomenon.")

Those of you who get to the biopsy stage, be forewarned. There is an appalling side effect of the internal harpooning. There will be blood present in the ejaculate for a few weeks, and not just trace amounts or even a few drops here and there. The first few post-biopsy orgasms revealed ejaculate that appeared to be mostly blood, but perhaps this was a trick of the mind. There was plenty of blood, though, especially in the first week after the biopsy. If a horror porn genre needs inspiration, this is sure to provide it. Less and less blood was present over the course of about four weeks until finally no blood was present. Also, the first few orgasms following the biopsy were a bit painful, as a result of the soreness associated with puncturing the rectal wall. The pain was not that great, of the kind that made me wince, certainly not sufficient to curtail the urge for release. Thus, there is the odd irony that the prostate is given time to heal before it is removed or irradiated.

Why did I need to climax so soon after such a procedure? Because I'm a guy, that's why. Seriously, any male knows that orgasm cuts down on anxiety, and I had a full share of angst during those days.

The specialist delivered the results directly to Doctor Fred, who called me into his office. By this time, some weeks after my initial visit to the walk-in clinic, long-suffering Debbie had flown in to be at John the patient's side. She was more alarmed than I was. Our recent lovemaking had taken on a fresh urgency that was bittersweet, as I understood that my sex life would be changed dramatically going forward.

Debbie and I sat across from Fred as he delivered the news, which was mixed. One of the probes had retrieved malignant tissue from two small tumors. Lab analysis of the sample reflected a Gleason score of 6. The Gleason scoring system measures two pieces of malignant tissue to determine the degree of differentiation in the cancer cells. Healthy cells are complete, almost round bodies that are quite distinct from one another. Partially malformed, pre-cancerous cells are called PIN (prostatic intraepithelial neoplasia). These cells are not malignant but are diagnostically uncertain, serving as a warning of cancer potential.

Under a microscope, cancer cells appear fused together in a shapeless mass. Unlike healthy cells, which live and die according to biological coding in their DNA, cancer cells do not die. Instead, they mutate, taking over nearby tissue and interrupting the proper functioning of the body parts under attack. It generally takes years before cancer in the prostate threatens to breach the gland's perimeter, but once it has breached the gland, its spread will typically accelerate, lessening the odds for a cure and complicating a patient's treatment options. And again, generally speaking, the younger one is afflicted, the more deadly the cancer. When oncologists refer to aggressive cancers they mean that the cancer replicates and takes over healthy tissue at a faster rate.

The various clinical stages of prostate cancer are described using several systems, but the two most common are designated ABCD and TNM. In the former system, A and B describe early phase cancers and C and D more advanced phases. In the TNM system, T stands for tumor, N for nodes and M for metastasis, which describes the disease's march from within the gland to the lymph nodes and beyond, to bones, lungs and other sites. There are several clinical books in print that cover this science if you wish to zone in on the specifics of your or a loved one's case.

The pathologist judges the "character" of the samples, assigning a Gleason score between 1 and 5 to each of the two pieces of tissue. Lower numbers indicate that the cancer cells are somewhat differentiated. Higher numbers indicate that an ugly, undifferentiated mass has formed. The two numbers are added together to result in a Gleason score of between 2 and 10. My score of 6 was in the intermediate range, but my cancer cells could mutate into a dangerous mass at any time. I needed treatment, and fast.

Thus, my cancer was subjectively described as moderately developed and somewhat aggressive. At the follow-up appointment in July 1999, Fred said that I needed to choose a course of action soon. He explained that even though my cancer had been growing slowly for years, it was now critical to get treatment within a couple of months. He is also an experienced surgeon, and said that if I chose surgery, I would be "made whole." I latched onto that phrase for all that it might promise. As someone acutely attuned to nuances of the English language, I gauged Fred's words one at a time, in segments, sentences and paragraphs and in their entirety, looking for possible death-dealing doublespeak. There was none. Vague language is unwelcome in such circumstances, so push your doctor for clear answers.

Fred tempered his statements with admonitions about the procedure, the recovery, and the fact that my sex life would be altered. I was calm as he said these things, as it occurred to me that, in many instances, Fred has had to deliver much graver news to men whose disease had progressed outside the gland. One of my musical heroes, Frank Zappa, had heard much graver news from Fred. Zappa died of the disease in December 1993. This must be the toughest part of Fred's job, although finding metastases when he opens a man up can't be fun, either.

Thinking of a breast cancer analogy, I asked Fred if a portion of the prostate could be removed, as opposed to all of it. No way, he said, explaining that the prostate operates as a whole and must be either irradiated from within, via seed implantation (called brachytherapy) or from the outside, via external beam radiation, or surgically removed altogether. I was too overloaded to ask any more questions at that point. I thanked Fred and retreated to the hallway, where Debbie broke down and hugged me tearfully. She was very upset. I was calm in a way I now figure the beachfront Nazis were when guarding Normandy's coast, watching as hundreds of Allied ships emerged from the June mist.

Never did I waver in my resolve to go the surgical route, as I had an image of the cancer relentlessly eating away at my insides, radiation notwithstanding. There was something especially sinister about some of my body's cells turning on me. Edgar Allan Poe story material. I wanted it out. I called a few people to get their input and one of these, Bob Milch, a doctor who had had the surgery himself, said he felt much better knowing that his cancer "was in a jar." I would not learn about my disease's confinement to the gland (or not) until later, after surgery. Fred had warned me that he wouldn't know my prognosis until I was opened up, and samples of surrounding tissue had been taken and sent to the lab. Waiting for definitive information was a repeatedly debilitating theme on my journey through the treatment maze. Not knowing almost drove me to another wing of the treatment facility, where the jackets have extra-long sleeves. I would much rather endure physical pain than live with a lack of critical medical information.

The next day, Fred and I agreed on a date for the surgery in early October 1999, about two and a half months away. That gave me enough time to face the music, as it were, to absorb thousands of pages of information about the disease, the treatment procedures, and the recovery process. I took time that summer to travel with Debbie to join my paternal cousins in the Outer Banks of North Carolina. I did not disclose my condition to them. One afternoon, I joined my cousins Neil and Mike for a round of golf, where I broke my driver halfway through the round. I was beyond tense. My reaction? More reading.

If a subject interests me, I can easily become obsessive about it, a trait Debbie knew could derange me. Left to my own devices, I was either going to become unhinged or become a medical research machine. She suggested I focus on putting my mind, if not at ease, at least at some intermediate level of acceptance. Once again, good advice, as I discovered months later that much of what I would learn was scary indeed. Readers who have advanced cases of prostate cancer have my deepest sympathy and I have corresponded extensively with some of them. To a man, they have been examples of courage. Perhaps foremost among them was a guy who was first diagnosed with a PSA of 1,000. More on him later. For years, he ran a very informative Web site, as he suffered from advanced disease, before succumbing in 2003. His e-mails to me had a tone of resignation I have come to acknowledge as part of thousands of sick guys' realities.

With reality churning my mind, sex took on poignancy much as I suspect occurs in wartime conditions. Tweaked by my angst and by Debbie's need to get me focused on what was important—love, a good attitude, and open lines of communication—I reveled in my highly functional sexual equipment, pushing my body to the limit. Any opportunity to put an erection to good use was heeded.

Eventually, Debbie had to return to New York City, to her job and to her delightful 17-year-old daughter. Over the coming weeks, the realization began to hit home, as reality grenades exploded in my head: I had cancer. Me. For whom the bell tolls. Though the bell of mortality was tolling weakly, I was determined to face the coming hardships with my head up. Yet much as I trusted Fred, I felt like snake eyes might tumble down on my operating table. The feeling of being cursed lingered from childhood.

Still, it took some weeks for the gravity of the diagnosis to sink in. One's life has a momentum that is suddenly stopped cold. Cancer. When the body turns on itself. I pictured gray blobs feeding off healthy pink tissue, a hostile takeover of the worst kind. Nightmares undermined my sleep. Yet I knew cancer could be beaten. It could be cut out of me and, if I were at all lucky, I would be cured. Some nights I wondered what had pushed me to accept Dr. Kevorkian's suggestion to have a PSA.

Was I slipping into self-pity? In my written pitch to the publisher of this book, I wrote: "The (prospective) author makes no claims to be a spiritual giant." To some degree, self-pity was at the core of perhaps two or three weeks of dark moods, but who under such circumstances would not suffer at least a mild bout of this ugliest defect of character? I would run from anyone who took such news with unflappable equanimity. Even as my own worst critic, I permitted myself some latitude for being angry that I had been chosen for a dark detour. And yet it was important that I do whatever it took to lift my spirits out of a "victim" framework. It proved healthier for me to get lost from time to time in the sense of wonder I had about science's role in the process. This feeling translated easily into gratitude for the fact that I was experiencing this malady at a time in medical history when something substantial could be done about it. Even 20 years ago, the blink of an eye in the timeline of man's development as a problem solver, my circumstances would have been much bleaker: no nerve sparing surgery would mean no erections, which in turn would mean . . . insert crude joke here.

I turned a bit glum for a while. Friends who knew my situation began to experiment with phrases and gestures toward me, trying to find a combination of supportive behavior that would bring me some comfort. As the day of the surgery approached, I kept thinking back to that day in June when Dr. Kuyt had delivered the news. Oftentimes, Debbie's smiles and tenderness could not cut through what I was feeling. At times, friction between us resulted in long silences. I wouldn't speak for days unless absolutely necessary. Ever a builder of psychological walls, I was at it again. Unanswerable questions held sway. "Why me?" was always good for a few fitful nights, which might give way to "You have been chosen to suffer this trial for some reason," which in turn led to "Accept the hand you've been dealt and play it as best you can." I understood, even while I was in the midst of it, that feelings of self-pity were a normal part of the grieving process, but still, acceptance did not come easy. Being picked as winner of the devil's lottery was another fleeting feeling, unnerving nonetheless, yet I do not believe in a God or a Devil who micro-manages our lives. At this point in the process, I was free to speculate on the best and worst of what was to come, for until my spirit settled down, I could not bring myself to call Fred about some of the concerns that were coming into focus. Fred had patients who were dying. He had better things to do. I still feel that way. I could always pick up another book, or cruise the Internet for validation or distractions.

I make a living with my imagination and my analytical abilities. Letting my mind roam over the bleak landscape of a future that might include impotence and incontinence, I had much motivation to put my original plumbing to full use. I flew to New York and made sure every session with Debbie was a 10-course feast, as I compensated for the capabilities that would soon be diminished. I am quite sure she was aware of these thoughts and impulses, even though we did not discuss the unfolding situation, although perhaps we should have. But of course there are times when words distract from the quality of the coupling.

I find it very hard to talk about my feelings for the simple reason that, like most American men, I was taught to keep my mouth shut unless I had something constructive to say. My problems were my problems, period, even as a kid. I am certain many men, even those who read this book full of warnings, will clam up and march through the diagnosis, the surgery and its aftermath with a hearty sternness. That said, or written rather, I hope the numbers of such men are fewer in this modern age. If ever there is a time to break out of the constrictive cultural mold American men live in, it is when faced with serious illness. Talk about it, with your wife, girlfriend, golfing buddies and, most of all, with your doctor. If your doctor won't talk until you feel like you're on an even keel, ready to move forward to the next phase of your process, get another doctor. If you are upset, that's as valid an emotion as any other. Millennia ago, the ancient Greeks perfected the dialectical method of finding truth. Talk it through. It is only cultural or personal hubris and ignorance that obstructs a more healing path.

If I suffered during the presurgery period more than was prescribed by the reality of the circumstances, I take responsibility for that. I do not think it is up to our partners to prompt or cajole emotions out of us. If you are uncomfortable talking about any aspect of the trial associated with prostate surgery and the aftercare process, then I suggest you find somebody or a support group and start talking. Keep in mind that if you or a loved one are to undergo a radical prostatectomy, the road for the next few years or so will be rocky, so put on your metaphorical hiking boots and get moving in the right direction.

At one point, between the time Fred confirmed my PSA and the biopsy confirmed the presence of cancer, I read a copy of Dr. Patrick Walsh's book *The Prostate: A Guide for Men and the Women Who Love Them*. Walsh is world-renowned as the key man in developing the nerve-sparing surgical technique that has saved many thousands of men from a life of impotence. His importance in the field cannot be overestimated. As a self-test in this area, ask yourself if, given the choice, you would rather be incontinent or impotent after surgery? Which group you fall into on this question may give you some clue as to how you might manage the emotional hurdles that recovery is sure to present. You are likely to have to deal with both issues to one degree or another. Walsh and his co-author are very careful in describing the debilitating aspects of advanced prostate cancer. One of the gloomiest is the symptomatology. "To put it bluntly, by the time a man has symptoms of prostate cancer, it's probably too late to cure it." And yet even this is not blunt enough get some of them to the surgeon's table.

In the years since I've had surgery, I've predictably had quite a few conversations with men age 45 and over, alerting them to the importance of the PSA test and the strong genetic factors involved in prostate cancer. Most men assure me that they have gone to their doctor, had the test, and are either clean, or doing something about an elevated reading. Yet there are a few guys I can think of who just will not deviate from what they feel is a righteously proud mindset. Call it the toothache syndrome.

This diabolical aspect of the disease will be addressed from time to time throughout this book, in a repeated effort to get to the hardest headed among "qualifying" readers. Even in this day and age, when the vast majority of men—and those who love them—are exposed to multiple channels filled with the latest medical information, denial still thrives. Even newspapers, that withering medium I love so much, feature the occasional article on prostate cancer. Older guys read newspapers. Why don't they get the message?

It would be great if I thought these mentions of the denial issue would suffice to get every affected reader off to treatment, but I know better. Thus, I apologize for the repetition in advance, especially to those less hard-headed. I dread the day a friend or acquaintance opens a conversation with any version of "John, I was having a little back pain, so I went to the doctor . . ." It will be too late for him, most likely, if that symptom reflects metastasis to the spinal column. Death by prostate cancer is one of the worst ways to shuffle off the mortal coil, so please, get your PSA tested and if you have cancer, waste no time getting treatment! Yes, it is an ordeal, but it is not that bad, certainly not as bad as it could be if you allow more time to pass.

This is not to say that staring down the specter of death is the way to go. Any influence that quells the inevitable fears that arise should be considered a gift from somewhere: God, Mother Nature, whichever source of strength works for you. In reflecting on this presurgery phase with the benefit of hindsight, there were a number of discussions I could have had with friends and loved ones to help ease the way to the scalpel. One of the issues that concerned me was that because most of Fred's patients were considerably older than me, they were not going to have their sexuality suddenly stolen from them by surgery. It is no secret that, for most men, by the time we are in our mid-50s our sex drive has decreased appreciably. This is not to say we become less interested in women—only that we become less driven biochemically to the series of thoughts, words and behaviors leading to sex and orgasm. Let's face it: Tireless twice-a-day sex is a game for young men.

However, I choose the word "stolen" with care, as that is what it felt like to me at the time. At age 46, I was still in robust shape libidinously and physically, with an urge to climax once a day on average. So sex, in one form or another, was still a big part of my daily routine. It may not bear scrutiny from some of my literary friends, but I had personified the cancer into a gun-wielding robber I was powerless against. It would steal my erections, steal my ejaculate, steal my sperm and hence my child-bearing capability . . . not that procreation was on any calendar associated with me. That goal had been scared out of me many years ago. I've never been mugged, but I can imagine I would not take it well.

A bigger question loomed: Would surgery steal my manhood? And what did that mean, exactly? Manhood was a collection of qualities, some physical, some psychological, some more difficult to quantify, such as the ethical qualities that shaped character and one's place in society. Intellectually, I know that manhood is measured in the quality of one's actions. But when threatened, it's human to give feelings their due. And if I felt my manhood was about to be taken away, would it be a theft in an irretrievable sense, or would there be something I could do about reclaiming it? Anxiety became the third player in my key relationship, accompanying

Debbie and me to bed, to the movies, while we were watching TV and she held my hand, often silently. She knew my mind was in a temporary black hole, but in the short term there was little more she could do about it.

Back in Hollywood, the content of available books on prostate cancer was decidedly redundant, which left me starving for first-person accounts and details of postsurgery intimacy. There wasn't very much out there on what it felt like to live without a prostate. Noted book editor Michael Korda had a book out, *Man to Man,* that I had hoped would touch upon all the intimate details I intended to cover. His book is appealing, but too polite. Even this book is too polite, but I'm hoping readers can read between the lines. For example, men are familiar with how anger can fuse with sexuality to create undesirable behavior. In the worst cases, crime results. In situations where a man is frustrated by difficulties in getting or maintaining an erection, anger from such circumstances may be expressed in a way that most women reject. There really is no way to describe in this book how some of my bouts with anger drove me to express my sexuality, but suffice it to say that there have been visceral moments, some of which I shared with my partner and some that I kept to myself. At least no one got hurt and appeasement was not required.

Firstly, I wanted to know what my chances were for achieving an erection postsurgery, and if there were none, how was a man expected to move through his days knowing he was impotent? Could I summon the courage to ask my lady if she'd stick by me if that were my future? Why would I have any expectation that she would stay with a sexually disabled partner, no matter how much she professed to love me? These were humbling questions. Unfortunately, I was not willing to accept any outcome other than one with positive results. Would I have written this book if I were impotent today? Not a chance. I'd have receded into the woodwork of my little beach community and led a life of complete anonymity.

A few weeks before the surgery date, October 5, 1999, it became plain to me that I had been relying too heavily on my sexuality to get through life's trials. My penis had been a crutch of sorts. A girlfriend once said that I used my penis like a kickstand. I took that remark to mean that rather than confront a problem within the context of possible practical solutions, I would use sex to prop myself up, distract myself from the often painful or merely annoying process of solving life's problems. At age 46, I became very uncomfortable with the idea that my character had a deep flaw that I was not interested in correcting. Living in Los Angeles did not help, as many men with careers in the arts enjoy success without becoming well-rounded individuals. Drugs, indiscriminate sex, and a general air of avoiding responsibility pervade Hollywood—and L.A. more generally. And yet cancer, taking me by the scruff of the neck, had already compelled me to seek a better balance in my life. Truth is, I do not like speaking. I would much rather listen. I am sure many readers will empathize with this attitude. I should add that I am a much better verbal communicator today than in the years prior to surgery.

Inevitably, my surgery date approached, the tick-tocking in my head growing louder. I still carried around a sense that I was cursed, so I didn't settle down dread-free until about three days prior to my prostate appointment with Fred. My fear of impotence had become considerable, much more so than my fear of incontinence. Other men I've spoken with since had the opposite concern. They were obsessed with the possibility of wearing disposable diapers or plastic bags for the rest of their lives. Both versions of these "what if?" scenarios are common, as our minds take flight in stressful circumstances. In fact, speaking for the surgical option, one starts over after surgery with no erectile ability and no ability to control urine flow. But I am getting ahead of myself.

Had I been, say, 76 years old at the time of the procedure rather than 46, I might have gone the other route and taken the chances attendant on radiation therapy. Or maybe I would have passed on treatment altogether. But at 46, I figured I had 30 more years of bouncing off the walls, sexually and otherwise, and I wanted to bounce around completely free of cancer, if possible. I would trust in Fred's analysis of my case and in the probability that I would rebound from the surgery to enjoy erections once again, albeit months later.

With the days counting down, there were a few tasks still ahead of me. One of the safeguards Fred recommended was that in the three weeks prior to surgery I should store two units of my own blood, in case the surgery was bloodier than anticipated. I complied with that recommendation, but thankfully, the surgery went smoothly, with a minimum loss of—to quote one of my favorite characters in movies, General Jack Ripper in *Dr. Strangelove*—precious bodily fluids.

(The actor who played Ripper, Sterling Hayden, was one of my favorite people, and I got to meet him once, when he came into the bookstore where I was working as a kid. He had tremendous physical presence, a man's man.)

Preparing one's mind and body for the ordeal of surgery and recovery is obviously critical to gaining some peace of mind during all phases of a complicated process. Among these preparations is meditation, which I highly recommend not just to prostate cancer patients, but to everyone. In California, where I live, such spiritual training is commonplace and will certainly spread throughout the country over time, once its benefits are more fully comprehended by the mainstream. So one afternoon that October, somewhat composed, I ejaculated for the last time, grabbed a few hours sleep and, bolstered by Debbie's compassion and concern, was off to the hospital that evening.

Three

SURGERY

7 A.M., October 5, 1999. I had been up for two hours, counting the holes in the ceiling panels. There were a few minutes of abject terror that subsided when I struggled successfully to take an objective perspective. I was just one of many thousands of guys who survived this ordeal. Gaining mental discipline is many times harder to attain when you do not have an active, positive role model in your life as a young kid, but I had quit drinking, and it had taught me how to make a life-altering decision and stick to it.

At last, a middle-aged orderly came to get me from my hospital room.

Lying on the gurney headed for surgery, I thought back to how I'd chosen the first doctor who seemed compassionate and sensitive to my fears about an uncertain future. It hadn't occurred to me then that everyone's future is uncertain. I had been in a dreamlike state when I walked into smiling Fred Kuyt's office and he sat back and appraised my dour mien for a few moments before speaking. It is very odd how one day you can be going about your everyday business with a circle of friends, family and business associates determining the course of your activities, and then the next day a perfect stranger sitting in front of you becomes, for a significant interval, the most important person in your life.

Just when I thought my mind would go, the friendly orderly wheeled me into the surgical wing. I calmed down immediately, because the waiting was over. As I was wheeled down the corridors, I recalled the last time Debbie and I had had sex. Our gyrations had been the last erotic extension of my "normal" body; neither of us knew if we would ever enjoy each other's bodies to the fullest again. For me, the most important psychological result of sex was the return to calmness afterwards, an elusive state of being for me. Two days previously, my mind had zigzagged up the psychic ramp toward climax, but there was a kind of kamikaze element to it. In the deepest recesses of my mind, I had known that, in a few seconds, the final ejaculation would in all likelihood bring an end to my ability to impregnate a woman, although there is an expensive urological procedure whereby the testes may be mined for sperm. I did not know of that medical trick at the time, nor did test tube pregnancies enter my thinking. It had definitely been my last "wet" orgasm. Even as I approached this moment, I wondered, Is this my last satisfying sexual episode? There was more than a little terror behind that final distortion of the psyche into the blinding vortex. And then, as they say, it was over.

Debbie had asked, "Are you all right?"

"I guess so," I'd said, and that about covered it.

We took a nap before I was to head over to the hospital to check in. On the ride over, I was quiet, resigned in a positive way to what was to happen. I reviewed my options one last time. Some years ago I had been involved in an effort to raise serious funds to start a company to research cryogenic methods of treating cancer. These involved either freezing or heating tumors to kill them. This was in the late 1970s, and the effort went nowhere, as potential investors were unconvinced, despite the parade of experts marshaled to testify to the concept's potential.

Back on the gurney, my thoughts moved on to radiation. If I had chosen either beam or seed type therapy, would I have been one of the lucky ones who would go on to live another 30 years untroubled by prostate cancer, or would it re-emerge in a year or two to herald the grave? I wasn't feeling like one of God's chosen children right about then, so I'd firmly settled on going ahead with the surgery. I realize that some readers will choose another option, watchful waiting, even though cancer is suspected or confirmed. I understand your reluctance, but please reconsider a more active course of treatment, as the longer you wait—

Another surgical method has emerged as a less invasive alternative to what I think of as the proven cut-open-like-a-fish approach, whereby an incision between the pubic bone and the navel presents the surgeon with his workspace. In the last few years, foremost in France, urologists have been treating prostate cancer by noncutting laparoscopic techniques, whereby a camera and operating tools are inserted down the penile opening via a catheter into the prostate. Surgery is performed almost by remote control. This procedure requires a great deal of additional training and extreme skill on the surgeon's part. It is just coming into vogue in the United States and promises shorter recovery times. More in vogue in the United States is a robotic technique where the body is accessed through five small incisions arrayed around the pubic area. It's good to have more options today, so be sure you understand them all before moving forward with your choice.

These newer techniques were not an option for me as I was geared up for the tried and proven method by which my doctor/friend Fred Kuyt had had so much success. In more than 95 percent of his procedures, out of a thousand or more, he had been able to spare the two nerve bundles that enable erections. Ninety-five percent was good enough for me; plus, I was young, which helped my odds. That was the primary concern for me. A life without erections? No, thank you. I was a depressive type as it was, even with my equipment working perfectly. Take that ability away and I'd be scrambling emotionally on a daily basis. I was keenly aware of how my maternal grandfather had ended his life, no doubt depressed.

Many men reading this book will make their choice of surgeon based on a less than thorough investigation. I empathize with that tendency, as I fought bouts of resignation in which I didn't care who did the surgery. At one point I was so ticked off I thought about doing it myself. Others will dawdle, which is equally dangerous, for time is of the essence when you have cancer in your prostate capsule. Please, gentlemen, be kind to yourselves and take the time to find the right doctor for the procedure. Choice of surgeon is not just related to rerouted plumbing. How your doctor interacts with you before and after surgery may either help or hinder your progress as you get acclimated to the changes wrought by the procedure. Make no mistake: The alterations to your sex life, and hence your emotional life, are significant. Certainly there are very good technical surgeons out there who are not good at communicating with their patients. This might not be a major issue for, say, correcting a hernia. The surgeon fixes the problem and you heal, and with luck a few checkups later you part ways. Not so with prostate surgery. At the very least, follow-up procedures continue for seven years, although doubtless many men do not follow through to that extent. If there are complications, of course the follow up will be more extensive, and for those needing hormone or chemotherapy, follow up may be open ended.

And then there's pride, a very tricky thing. Some say it's always a bad thing; others claim it's a necessary adjunct to self-esteem. Certainly, pride can be a vicious thing. In my case, pride was a reflection of three facts: One, in my mid-40s I could still achieve and maintain erections with the rigidity and reliability of a teenager; two, I was hard-wired to derive primary satisfaction from the satisfaction of my sexual partners; and three, what wavering self-esteem I had was accumulated largely through acceptance from women, which set me as far apart from my father as possible. When my father was in the final stages of alcoholism, he became impotent, which transmogrified into sexual identity issues that devastated me as a young man. I would prove I was the virile male he was not, and moreover, I would never abuse women the way he had abused my mother. So, yes, I was, as they say, compensating for another's failures, which is predictable human behavior. One can infer from these three psychological components that I would have a tough time with the after-effects of surgery, which were guaranteed to reduce my effectiveness as a boudoir crusader.

In the short term, though, only one sentence of Fred's had registered with any permanence: "You will be made whole." Even so, as a mad dog mangles a rag doll, over the intervening months self-pity had threatened to rip me asunder when I was not careful to stay centered and grateful for the many gifts I had been given.

Sometimes gratitude extended to the basics: Arms and legs, a sharp mind, good friends and great general health. I also held on to some gratitude for having had a clear full-body CAT scan, except for the two malignant tumors in my prostate. Muddled as my thinking was, I could begin to imagine what it might be like for other men less fortunate.

(I should mention that when they inject the iodine solution into you for a body scan, which they perform to get a baseline reading of your entire system, there are a brief few seconds when the body convulses from the introduction of this very foreign substance. The effect passes quickly, but it is alarming nonetheless.)

In many traditional families it is the wife's task to address medical issues, including choosing doctors and making appointments. So be it. Gather as much practical information as possible, but perhaps someone in your family other than you is better at that task. Maybe a son or daughter is a wizard on the Internet. Many readers will be reluctant to ask questions of doctors because they do not want to "bother" them. Prostate cancer is a life or death matter and warrants any prospective caregiver's complete attention, once they have been engaged to discuss your case. Certainly it helps if you arrive with a good amount of foreknowledge on the subject. Don't settle for a prepared drone of an explanation. At a minimum, be familiar with the Gleason scale, the system for gauging the severity of a cancer's spread and the type of cancer that is present. Some prostate cancers grow very slowly and can linger undetected for decades. In fact, very often men die of old age or other maladies before the cancer grows and spreads to become life threatening. At the other extreme, some prostate cancers grow quickly and can kill their hosts within months. Most cancer types fall somewhere in the middle, as did mine. And yet I recall a local fundraiser for the widow of a guy who died of the disease at 35. The question is: How willing are you to leave room for doubt, second-guessing and error in this once-in-a-lifetime circumstance?

Make lists. Please do not rely on memory, as the propensity to forget well-intended and even crucial information is strongest early in the process. Even if carrying a written list of questions seems ridiculous to you, do it. Another issue is procrastination, which was an issue for me, as someone who is not only self-employed, but who also works alone for the most part.

Once diagnosed, I had wanted to buy some time before the surgery, if for no other reason than to enjoy my "whole" body for as long as was practicable. But once I had read up on the disease, I only needed to sit still for a minute and imagine the cancer creeping out of the prostate capsule and into the neighboring lymph nodes and beyond into the pelvis and wherever. Self-chastened, I agreed to a minimum delay of only a few months from diagnosis to surgery. Had it not been for the biopsy and the healing required from it, I would have agreed to have the surgery the next day. Or perhaps I would have asked Fred to take it out in his office with a letter opener during our July meeting.

It takes a few months to heal from the nasty, hollow needle that takes prostate tissue samples, so four months passed between diagnosis and surgery. It was an unpleasant wait. As noted earlier, in the intervening summer months I "vacationed" on North Carolina's Outer Banks with some of my cousins, who had rented a huge house for a couple of weeks. The stress got to me on the golf course, where I was unable to hit the ball cleanly. At one point, gripping the driver like a baseball bat, I broke it and quit for the day. Months later, when my cancer and surgery became known to my extended family, my cousin Neil asked me if I had known about the malignancy during our vacation. I admitted I had, which put my brooding in a context that made sense to him, and to me.

Picture a bald, six-foot two-inch maniac, like Khrushchev banging his shoe, standing before you in an auditorium as I deliver these words. Tough guys! I strongly recommend that you soldier blithely on with an "I'll get to it" attitude only if you admit to those who love you that you have a death wish. If it makes more sense, follow through not for yourself, but for those who love you. Deal with your cancer now, because nothing is more important than your health. Or do you want to spend the remainder of your days concerning yourself primarily with pain management?

Make no mistake, for most of my adult life after I gave up drinking in 1984, I was one of those men who took his overall health for granted; if it didn't hurt, I must be all right. Yet, for years, the cancer was slowly growing in me. Fred figured 10 years or more. My guess is it was triggered by my getting clean from booze, which so changed my body chemistry that I became allergic to animals for the first time in my life, and ever after. (It kills me that I cannot have a dog, even a hypoallergenic one.)

Given the reality that prostate cancer doesn't hurt until it's too late, perhaps you're at the point where you've recently had a general physical administered by your family doctor. Everything is fine except for your PSA test, which came back elevated, above a 4.0 reading. It would be easy to procrastinate at this point with "I'll get to it" rationalizations. Your family doctor should be exhorting you to see a urologist immediately, especially if your PSA is into double digits or higher. I reiterate: my PSA was about 7.0 when I was diagnosed. Had I not had that physical in the spring of 1999, perhaps a few years would have passed and the cancer might have metastasized throughout my body. Enough beating you over the head with warnings. By now you're either with it or you're not. I'll put my shoe back on.

Another point to consider is, how well do you really know your family physician? If you're going to take a doctor's recommendation regarding a urologist/surgeon, you must be sure your generalist is well-informed about the disease, current treatments, and the importance of communication in the preparation/surgery/follow-up equation. Before investigating further, ask your doctor how he knows the urologist he is recommending. (Please pardon the male pronoun "he"; I use it for expediency only and because I assume that the vast majority of doctors older men go to are men themselves.) If he met him at a convention a month ago that's different than if he's known him professionally for 20 years. In the latter case, call the recommended urologist's office and ask about his approach to prostate cancer. He may favor radical prostatectomy or radiation or some combination of treatments. Note that nearly every practitioner will offer you a biased perspective. As a professional, each specialist must "profess" adherence to his preferred medical principles based on the belief system constructed during his medical school education and as a resident physician. You are very unlikely to find a urologist who offers surgery and radiation as equal options. He will most likely mention the alternatives to his favorite course of treatment, and then present a persuasive case for his specialty. This is another reason why it pays to educate yourself before engaging specialists in discussion. It is important to be comfortable with your choice. No one else will be living with it as intimately as you.

If the biopsy is positive and you have cancer, take it slow, and pay close attention to what your urologist says in your follow-up meeting. If your doctor is a good communicator, you are likely to get a somewhat personalized education about not just your diagnosis, but also statistics on men who have had cancers of similar type and aggressiveness. Listen up! Or at least bring your spouse or significant other along to listen for you. This can be a very trying time and it is normal for your mind to wander off into denial or shock. In my case, what Dr. Kuyt was telling me went in one ear and maybe 90 percent went out the other. All I heard was "You will be made whole." Debbie retained the rest.

Somewhere in the part about being made whole, Fred said that if the disease is caught early, as in my case, a guy is going to want the best surgeon possible to take it out. And by "it" I am referring to the prostate gland, which is completely removed when it is cancerous, no matter how small the tumor. Hence the term "radical prostatectomy," as opposed to partial—there is no such thing. I had hoped they could cut out the malignancy and leave the gland somewhat intact, but it doesn't work that way.

The idea that I would need to lose the entire gland upset Debbie tremendously. Looking back, I suspect she was drawing a parallel to the choices addressed by women with breast cancer. It must be one thing for a woman to have a lump removed and another thing to have the entire breast removed. Thus, in the surgical realm, it would seem to vary from person to person, but at some point a procedure becomes severe enough to permanently alter a patient's sense of self. Certainly, as I write these words years after surgery, I can safely say that my identity has been altered significantly and permanently. In fact, my main motivation in writing this book is to provide readers with details about these permanent changes and how I cope with them. For women, I would think that whereas a lumpectomy is very much less likely to induce permanent psychic change, a radical mastectomy crosses a psychological threshold. Even though most women who undergo a radical procedure do not leave the hospital without reconstructive surgery, the simple fact that cancer has encroached on one's life may present the widest, darkest barrier to be crossed.

So consider that if your urologist is very good, he will be much more than a competent scalpel-wielding technician. He will also be a quasi-psychiatrist, skilled in getting his patients to talk freely about their fears, their moods, and their futures over the course of years of treatment. This is not to suggest that practical concerns about your urologist's ability and professional experience do not take precedence over a touchy-feely patient management style. It is of course paramount that your surgeon have a stellar surgical track record. These records include the percentage of patients who live cancer free for at least five years, and the percentage of patients who retain the two nerve bundles that enable erections. I would avoid any surgeon who is not forthcoming with his professional statistics in these two areas, or run from one who has a less than 90 percent success rate in either of these two categories.

Once you're comfortable with your choice of surgeon, focus on what he is about to do. His tasks include excising the gland—and hopefully all of the cancer—and rerouting the urethra and blood vessels that were feeding blood to the gland. As detail-obsessed patient as I was, even I did not have sufficient curiosity to find out how many blood vessels would be cut and how they would be either tied off or rerouted. I had to draw the line somewhere. Suffice it to say it took Dr. Kuyt about four hours to perform the procedure on me. At least I didn't need the two units of blood that had been stored for me.

In terms of surgery in general, radical prostatectomies are routine procedures in the medical theater, yet each one involves complicated work by the surgeon, no matter how many he has performed. You are the star in your own operating-room drama and there are no shortcuts in performing a standard RP. Thus, it would also be good to know how many procedures your doctor has performed. If the number is fewer than 20 or so, consider someone with more experience.

Secondly, even when you're certain your surgeon meets the technical criteria, strongly consider how you can play a role in optimizing his ability as a communicator. You have a job to do, too. There are ways to ask questions that contribute to the process and there are fear-driven questions that may put a rift between you and this suddenly key person in your life. Certainly, your doctor is not going to expect a cheerful demeanor as you gather information, yet you do not want to come across as a handful either, let alone a lunatic. A controlled, even tone when you ask questions will go a long way, as will a trip to the library or bookstore, to prove that you're taking a proactive role in the process. If you are shy about discussing the physical and mental aspects of sex, now is a great time to get over it, or at least open up a bit. You don't want to be plagued years later with a list of "what ifs."

No matter how willing you are to investigate the details of the surgery and post-surgery process, the message is clear. The more you know about your case, the better. Nonetheless, there will be many of you who prefer to stick your heads in the sand about the whole thing. Men who do that are going to have a much tougher time in recovery. It has been tough enough for me over the years, and I consider myself very well informed.

Of course, the mental aspects of recovery linger long after the eight-inch vertical scar has healed. Put yourself in your urologist/surgeon's white smock for a moment. He is likely a confident professional, with many years and scores of procedures to draw from. Each patient who has cancer falls into one of several categories, but basically patients fall into three camps: (1) the prostate cancer is caught early, confined to the gland, and prognosis for complete recovery is very good; (2) the prostate cancer is more developed, and it is suspected to have migrated outside the gland, which would generate an uncertain prognosis until the surgeon operates, makes an onsite assessment, takes samples of nearby lymph nodes and through follow-up testing, determines the extent of the cancer's spread, and: (3) the prostate cancer has definitively spread beyond the gland into the lymph nodes and perhaps the spinal column and pelvic bones, the most likely targets of metastasis. In this last instance, the prognosis is generally poor, and the patient's life expectancy may be several years or in some cases, months.

This book is predominantly for men whose disease is confined to the gland. Insofar as I did not undergo radiation or hormone therapy, I cannot share such experiences in this limited memoir. In every case, how the news is delivered is critical to the patient's state of mind going forward. I often consider how Fred Kuyt has had to deliver terrible news to men whose cancer has spread throughout their bodies, as a diagnosis of metastasized prostate cancer is almost uniformly grim. Even in cases like mine, where the cancer is confined to the gland, no particular outcome is certain. The urologist must tailor his verbiage very carefully. Words should be chosen with surgical care.

A variation on an old joke comes to mind. A man with a high PSA enters his urologist's office, expecting biopsy results. The gorgeous receptionist asks him to take a seat. Later, in the doctor's office, the doctor says, "I have good news and bad news. Which first?"

"The bad news," says the glum patient.

"The bad news is you have prostate cancer," says the doctor, and the patient looks up hopefully. "The good news is, right after you leave my office, I'm going to bend the receptionist over a chair and screw her silly."

I like this joke because it lays bare the component of self-pity in this situation. The perception is that others may go on about their sexual exploits as normal, virile males, while those who have suffered an RP may be designated as the droop troop, patrolling the bleak byways of the lonely and misbegotten. But the best part of the joke is the patient's expectation that the good news applies to him. Such is man's lovable propensity to hope for the best. I like this quality in us.

No matter the prognosis, the C-word is likely to send most men into a tailspin, and this is entirely normal. But we need to rebound and face the future, come what may, and a compassionate doctor should be second only to a life partner as a source of comfort and encouragement. If you are going it alone, look for support groups in your area. Your doctors may have suggestions as well, and the Internet is a lifeline, too. And don't count women out as helpers. A good woman will be at your side if you are open and honest about all aspects of your life.

In this age of HMOs and related forms of commercialized medicine, one cannot presume that nearly all doctors are compassionate. Surely many readers have been fortunate to have been tended to by warm human beings who happen to be physicians. But there are plenty of greedy body mechanics out there, especially in the United States, where the money to be made has enticed dispassionate technicians into the medical fold. I truly hope readers can identify such people when they encounter them. Moreover, as reprehensible as it is, as of this writing the United States does not have a national health care program, though I am hopeful that President Obama will do something meaningful about that, perhaps in his second term, after the economy has been righted. If we can bail out banks and auto companies, why can't we bail out our sick citizens? This shameful situation does not mean that you have to take the first doctor your HMO-restricted plan offers you. I have heard stories from men about how their doctors delivered the news. Some of these details are almost as horrifying as the disease itself. One man who had an advanced case was met with these first words: "Well, Jim, you'd better get your affairs in order." If I had a terminal case of prostate cancer and my doctor chose that sentence as his opener, he'd need to get his affairs in order, too.

Let's back up a bit, to October 1999. Check-in to the hospital had gone smoothly, and soon enough I had been wheeled into the private but stark room. Debbie had brought a magazine to read as I settled in on one of those adjustable hospital beds designed by sadists masquerading as industrial engineers. It was early evening, about 12 hours before the surgery, which was scheduled for 7 A.M. the next morning. I watched TV for a while, and then Debbie left to go back to my place. She had been ready to stay the night with me, curled up in a chair in my room, but I was convinced she had done enough for one day so I thought it best for her to sleep in a real bed and return the next day, when I was likely to be an emotional mess. As she was leaving, she had one of those looks on her face that said: "I don't think I'm doing the right thing . . ."

Then the nurse returned with the potion that would clear out my bowels several hours before surgery. This is necessary to minimize the chances of infection in case the surgeon accidentally cuts into the intestine. Septicemia can kill you, so expect to be loaded up on antibiotics after both the biopsy and the surgery. Make sure you inform all medical personnel if you have any drug allergies. If you don't know, say so, so your doctor can watch for adverse reactions.

Insofar as it's necessary to drink about a half gallon of the bowel cleanser (I'm exaggerating, but only a little), I took one sip just to acclimate my palate. It was vile, the worst sludge I'd ever tasted, and as a recovering alcoholic, I have a very high threshold for "vile." You'd think that science, having put a man on the moon 30 years earlier, could create a fruit-flavored concoction to do this job, but apparently not.

Thankfully self-preservation has rejected any specific sensory memory of the taste of that vile liquid, but suffice it to say that I had a very tough time getting the stuff down, gagging over and over. I was only able to drink about two-thirds of the swill, and at one point I threatened a nurse who kept insisting I drink more. All I did was glare at her, really, but it was enough to send her scurrying for a supervisor, who came in and said "Mr. Hallenborg, you must drink all of the fluid if—"

"You drink it! I'd rather die!" I snapped. It was that bad. I have a history of ulcers, so maybe the witch's brew they were feeding me would sit better with most folks; I don't know. Maybe by the time most of the readers of this book have surgery, they'll be given a lemon-flavored version of the stuff. I certainly hope so.

By the time I sent the supervising nurse packing, it was about 1 or 2 A.M. I was alone, and the world started to get very small. I realized I'd been an idiot for sending Debbie away. I lay back in bed, counted the holes in the ceiling tiles, watched TV. Losing the calm I had been feeling for most of the day, I so wished my lady were there to rub my brow, get me a cold compress, fix me with a smile. I buzzed the nurse, had her shift my bed into the horizontal position and somehow got some sleep, which was dreamless and not aided by drugs.

I awoke at 6:15 A.M. The clock on the wall seemed to have stopped. A nurse looked in, smiled, went about her duties. I was developing a mild headache. At 6:45 I had an episode of stark terror that I wouldn't wish on anybody. I saw the whole event in black and white, and became convinced that something was going to go terribly wrong. I could feel the little boy inside me, always raging, looking for a way out of the double bind (can't fight, can't flee) he felt he was trapped in. It was tough to get the adult in me to calm the raging kid down, to shut him up. I must have exhausted myself, for suddenly I glanced up and there was a middle-aged orderly, standing over me with a tired smile, ready to wheel me to surgery.

Instantly, my mood turned around and I was eager to get on with it. The clock-watching had been killing my spirit. Just outside the operating room, there were a few other patients waiting their turn to go under the knife for a variety of reasons. This was a humbling moment. I realized that if any one of those patients had been a child who started crying, I would break down crying myself. Adult emotions I could handle, so I looked around and met the worried gazes of kindred spirits meeting once in untoward and expectant circumstances.

There was a pretty blonde woman in her 20s who seemed embarrassed to be seen without make-up, or maybe it was something else. She smiled weakly. I was about to ask what she was in for, but there was something dire beneath her smile, so I let it go. I said "See you in recovery" instead, and she smiled back but didn't speak.

Further down the hallway was an older guy who kept sitting up and looking around, much to his nurse's consternation. I laughed, and he could tell I appreciated his Do-not-go-gentle-into-that-bright-OR feistiness. He kept swatting at his nurse as she tried to get him to lie still. Finally, an anesthesiologist arrived to put the old guy under, and he was wheeled inside.

I could hear a woman crying softly around the corner. I pushed against the wall to move my gurney so I could see her. She was in her early 40s, tired, elegant, scared. She was one of those people one feels comfortable around right away. Call it the texture of her dignity. She sighed, acknowledging my attention.

"A female thing," she said before I could ask.

"Prostate surgery," I replied.

She laughed. "That about covers it!" After a long pause, she added, "I never had any kids," in a way that made me feel both that she had wanted several and that, if we hurried, maybe we could make one just then.

"Me neither," I said, hardly a champion for the subject.

"Good luck!" she said, as she was wheeled in.

"You, too," I said, glad not to have any more time to ruin the moment with a misplaced, over-reaching joke. Just like me to flirt in such a gloomy situation.

Finally, Fred's anesthesiologist, whom I suspected also ran a hardware store, given his casual air, came out to see me. "I'm going to give you a little something to take the edge off before we put you under."

Yeah, right. For the record, don't be fooled when they tell you this. He put me under right there, out in the hallway, with a shot in the butt. Then I suppose—because I was out like a light—Fred Kuyt proceeded to slice and cut and tie off and shunt and whatever else he did in there, for the next three or four hours. I didn't dream, or if I did, I had no recall of dreaming while I was in the OR. Cut to me out in the hallway again where, through considerable delirium, I could just make out Debbie's pretty, expectant face and Fred's benevolent smile. I don't recall reaching for Debbie's breasts just then but I was told later that that is what I did in my anesthetic haze. She observed my groping and said "You're fine, honey!" I have learned not to trust the word "fine" coming from any woman, so I looked to Fred, who nodded in a way that brought me much relief.

"Everything went great," Fred said. "Very little blood loss, everything nice and neat. We saved the nerve bundles."

That was the best possible news. I'd once worked for a talented man who had had prostate surgery in the 1960s, when there was no nerve-sparing procedure. He was a generally genial guy, but had a gruff streak and, like me when I knew him, he drank every day. Enough said. Would I have gone back to drinking myself to death if those nerves bundles hadn't been spared? Good question, and I still don't know the answer.

Back in my room I was delirious, mostly from relief. The mortality rate from prostate surgery is very low, but I had been feeling very unlucky lately. Debbie milled about, making sure I had what I needed—sports on TV, a book or two, magazines, water. A nurse wheeled in an IV stand holding a morphine drip. Once she had me hooked up, she gave me a microphone-shaped gizmo with a button on it so I could self-administer a dose of the powerful painkiller whenever I needed it. The dosage was regulated, of course, and with my history as an addictive type, I made sure I kept the dose well below the permitted maximum.

My fears that the morphine would get me high were unfounded. It did not, not at all. Rather, it simply kept the pain at bay, so that I could begin moving around a little. My memory of the hours just after surgery is fuzzy, but I recall being annoyed at the catheter and the plastic bag I was urinating into, which prompted a feeling of helplessness that would grow worse before long. Nonetheless, I slept well that first post-op night.

The next day, the day nurse instructed me to get out of bed and begin walking around, morphine drip and catheter apparatus attached. Adding to the discomfort, the surgical incision, an eight-inch vertical slash just to the left side of and down from my navel to the pubic bone, itched some, as did the catheter, but I was determined to get moving.

I shuffled along out in the hallway, under a nurse's care, not caring if my butt was hanging out. (I have been told I have a nice butt, and at one time I took to promoting it as the Globes of Sweden. Word should reach you soon.) It was odd to be both lucid and pain-free, as the morphine was so much more effective than any pain pill I had ever taken. Toward the end of the first day I was encouraged to shuffle around solo, which I did, perhaps to excess, to keep my mind and body occupied. There was a very pretty nurse working the night shift, and her white uniform fit very snugly.

Her "I'm unattainable" attitude and clinging white uniform prompted my first post-op thoughts of sex as she sauntered away from me, her confidence and taut bottom triggering the familiar "want" response in the back of my brain. Yet the physical act of sex seemed so remote at that moment that I worried I would be relegated to a scrap heap of aging eunuchs. I pictured a very sad retirement community in Florida full of them. Self-pity does not foster sympathy, but it was a small part of my process, and I own up to it.

My primary real concern was the biopsy of the lymph nodes adjacent to the prostate. These had been removed for inspection as a matter of course, for although my PSA score was low compared to most men whose cancer had migrated outside the prostate capsule, there was still a chance that cancer could be found in the nodes. Note in Fred's preface that he writes of a young man with a fatal case who had a PSA of 1.9 at diagnosis. There is no guarantee that a particular man's body will produce prostate specific antigen in response to the presence of cancer. If any of my lymph nodes did turn out to be cancerous, I had radiation treatments to look forward to in an even more uncertain future.

By the end of Day Two of my hospital stay, I was moving around the hallway quite well, pleased with my rapid recovery, cajoling the nurses, encouraging less ambulatory patients. Then they took the morphine away. I awoke on the third morning post-op, tried to turn over and groaned loudly enough to prompt a nurse to check in on me. I assured her I was okay, and she smiled, saying it was time I learned to heed my body's signals as to its true condition. Suddenly, every movement caused a great deal of pain. I was given the painkiller Toradol intravenously for a while, then transferred to some pills—Vicodin I believe—but it was candy compared to the morphine. Debbie was dismayed to see me in pain, but I assured her I just needed to learn to slow down. She knew even then that impatience would be the biggest hurdle to my recovery. She was ready to crack me over the head if I got out of line.

Then Fred arrived to inform me that the nodes were clear of cancer. No radiation for me. I was overwhelmed with gratitude, both to Fred and to Debbie, and also to Dr. Kevorkian, who had had the foresight to include the PSA test in my physical exam months earlier. Fred also told me to slow down, and to follow the nurses' instructions about what I could eat and drink. He knew I was very poor at taking instructions, much less orders. To get me to do anything, it's best to suggest indirectly or to disguise instructions within a larger framework of information. My friends all know how to do this, and Fred was becoming one of them.

Eventually, I recommenced perambulating around the hospital hallway. Each step triggered a wince and a long intake of breath. I was starting over. It became clear that the road to recovery would be uphill. Exhausted by a half-hour tour around the nurses' station and by too much anticipation of an uncertain future, I fell into a coma-like sleep.

I had been explicit with friends about visiting me in the hospital. I wasn't comfortable seeing people. My old buddy Dennis dropped by, as did an acquaintance, a cute and bubbly lady named Jennifer, whom I knew from A.A. She and I became friends later on, though she has disappeared from my life today. Her visit went well, though, as she has the kind of upbeat energy that cannot fail to raise one's spirits. I found out later she had a brain tumor and was in denial. I hope she's okay.

When I was three days off morphine and cruising along on a low dose of Vicodin, Fred signed me out of the hospital. Urinary catheter firmly attached to my leg, I wobbled to the hospital garage and a rental car. I was folded in and Debbie drove us home. There was to be no driving for me for a while, doctor's orders. We didn't want to risk pulling the catheter out prematurely, which would mean I would never be continent again. Unshowered for days, I felt grimy, tired and stoop-shouldered, my dour personality hidden under a cloaking haze of shock and medication, like the Aqualung character in the Jethro Tull song. Time to settle my catheter, urine bag and shell-shocked psyche at home, in familiar surroundings. Oh, and don't forget the painkillers!

Four

CONVALESCENCE

Somebody once came up with a great line: If you want to hear God laugh, tell him your plans. I thought I had a failsafe system in place for when I returned home to recuperate. First, Debbie would tend to me before returning to New York, and then a friend would take over, when she could, get me groceries and make sure I hadn't cracked my skull open en route to the bathroom. But cancer puts fear into people, and I discovered that one's close friends are no exception. Debbie administered her usual gracious care, and her patience with me was inspiring. My other friend, however, was nowhere to be found once Debbie returned to New York. So the message is, be sure you pick your caregivers carefully, lest they get spooked. The Big C has such unpredictable effects on people, whether they're the ones who have it or not.

Cancer's effects often extend into social situations, as one might guess. You will find people act strangely for one reason or another whenever cancer is in the room. One guy I know, a highly educated misfit, is a proud wearer of $50 washable, reversible suits. He was at an event where a cancer sufferer's wife was discussing her husband's fears. "It's only recently he's been able to say the 'c' word," she said. The misfit intoned, "Yeah, I couldn't say c*nt out loud for the longest time either." Expect surprises from surprising sources.

Back in my place in the Hollywood Hills, I settled into bed as my personal Florence Nightingale set about taking care of me in her efficient manner. Debbie is so full of love it is humbling. My memory of those initial postsurgical days at home is fuzzy, as the pain pills were more effective at fragmenting my awareness than they were at alleviating pain, which was intolerable only when I tried to use my stomach muscles. As they say back in New York, forget about it. A method akin to logrolling worked best when getting out of bed, as the urinary catheter kept necessary excursions to the bathroom to a minimum. Yes, I fell down a few times.

In case you haven't had the pleasure of experiencing a urine catheter, let me describe it to you. It consists of a plastic tube running from your bladder down your urethra, through the penile opening down to a urine collection bag strapped to your leg. For the first several weeks after surgery, you will have no control over when you go, nor how much. You wake up after surgery with this thing inside you and it absolutely cannot be removed if you are to heal properly, so get used to it as quickly as you can. The best thing to do is just embrace the reality and be grateful. You could be much worse off. However, heavy grumbling is encouraged. The bag will fill up when you sleep and you will learn to empty it on a schedule that will evolve over a week or two. And keep in mind this charming side effect that I had not been warned about. My scrotum became extremely swollen, ballooning to a size that would be appropriate on a male a much larger species, say a bull or perhaps a rhino. It became an unwieldy, very large handful, to put it mildly. I do not recall how long it took to recede, perhaps a month or so. Insert more bad jokes here.

Soup was the main diet staple in those early post-op days, which was fine by me. I didn't feel like eating. Debbie ran errands in her rental car while I watched TV and tried to read a little. All very mundane stuff, but the simple routine allowed my head to settle so I could begin to make the psychological adjustments I knew would either make or break me in long-term recovery. On the one hand, the surgery was behind me, as evidenced by the ugly eight-inch scar with its thick black sutures. On the other hand, I kept wondering, would I ever get another erection? Forget the Holy Grail, people; this was more important. Would I be one of the unfortunate few who never rid himself of the catheter? If so, could I summon the strength of character to live in a positive way that reflected an acceptance of one or more permanent infirmities? I thought so, but could not be sure.

Underneath the effects of the Vicodin, anxiety about sex emerged. I began fidgeting and talking about anything that came into my head. Debbie put up with my rambling, perhaps because, generally, I'm not much of a talker. When I'm in writing mode, I can go days without speaking, and it doesn't occur to me that anything odd has transpired. Silence is gold usually, platinum on occasion. But now, a bit bored with myself, I called a few friends, some of whom came to visit, including an actor friend, Dewey, whose eyes went wide at the Frankenstein-type stitches that traced the surgical cut above my groin. He was in his 30s at the time, so I spared him my usual warning about getting his PSA checked. I'll say something to him in a couple years, when he's 50.

Over the first two postsurgery weeks my routine did not vary much. I awoke, emptied the urine bag, took a shower, ate some cereal, went back to bed, read or watched TV (for exciting TV, nothing could compare to the North Hollywood bank shootout that had occurred two years earlier), slept, woke, read some more, took some phone calls, ate soup for dinner, read or watched TV, slept. Getting dressed with the catheter bag attached involved contortions and sliced up pajamas. My body ached and the stitches itched. Very exciting stuff. Plus, I had a rubber sheet on the bed. Of all the things about those early days I don't miss, that has to be one of the main ones.

Then a crisis occurred. Two weeks into recovery, I got up in the middle of the night to get some juice and passed out on the kitchen floor. Luckily, I didn't fall on the catheter bag. Debbie was awakened by the thud of me hitting the tiles. She managed to get me back into bed, but I was very, very weak. In the morning we packed up again and went back to the hospital, this time to the emergency room. I barely made it into a lobby chair under my own power. (This sort of thing will not apply to nearly every reader. I only include it as information about possible postsurgical consequences and medications. Make sure to heed any warnings your body gives you.)

It was quickly determined that I was bleeding internally, from a duodenal ulcer. I was somewhat surprised, but given that I had had ulcers when I was 17, at least there was a precedent. I had been under a lot of pressure prior to surgery, having finished up a large writing project literally the day before the procedure. Other matters had been weighing on me as well, so my stress level was high both right before and right after surgery.

When I had ulcers as a kid, they hurt. I had been doubled over in my hospital bed, unable to find a comfortable position. So this time, because there was no pain, just weakness, I didn't recognize the more dangerous symptoms of simply and painlessly bleeding out. One exacerbating medication may have been the Toradol, which is contraindicated for a patient with an history of ulcers. But I hadn't had an ulcer in almost 30 years, so I doubt I'd mentioned it on any of the forms I filled out for Fred.

There was much running around in the ER until they got me stabilized. Then the ER staff knocked me out and sent me to surgery, where the internist on call, Dr. Soraya Ross, tended to the angry puncture in my intestinal tract. She's a fine doctor, too, and I see her every couple of years for check-ups. The hole, just south of my stomach, was accessed through a thick tube down my nose. This procedure is no picnic, either. I needed several units of blood and came to in a private room on an upper floor of the hospital.

Debbie was there, of course, holding my hand, with a look on her face that said "What am I going to do with you?" I was in low-level shock by this point, the accumulated experiences of the last few weeks having caught up with me. A nurse gave me a sedative and I said good-bye to Debbie yet again. She headed back to my place as I watched the TV drone on softly.

It was 2:46 A.M. on October 16 when the Hector Mine earthquake struck, the biggest to hit the area in some years. It registered 7.1 on the Richter Scale, but thankfully its epicenter was way out east in the desert, far from L.A. A 7.1 quake centered close by might have sent me flying across my hospital room. Despite the distance from the epicenter, though, my hospital bed on wheels started rolling around the room. It was most disconcerting and somewhat funny. When the motion stopped, I used an electrical cord as a lifeline to pull the bed back near the bedside table with the phone, so I could call Debbie at my place. It was her first earthquake, and she didn't know what to do with herself. My neighbors had congregated out in the courtyard, in case a severe aftershock—or bigger main shock—weakened the apartment building's structure. Fortunately, the worst had passed and the next day I was headed home, yet again.

Take Two. I resumed my routine of shuffling around the apartment, not looking forward to the day Debbie had to leave. But this time I was much, much weaker from losing so much blood. Debbie had a job in New York, and a daughter to take care of, but by the time she needed to leave, I was moving around pretty well, spirits raised. She and I had a tearful, mostly joyful parting, and then I was on my own for the next few months, although I had a lot of help in the endearing form of Eleanor, an angel, as the song goes, of the first degree.

Eleanor is a singer/songwriter with nifty tattoos and a mischievous smile. She is one of those people with so much talent she hardly knows which direction to take. She can sing, act, write, etc., and she is mad cute and charming as well. Best of all, there is a deep warmth about her that anyone can respond to; I'm very grateful she helped me when I was somewhat incapacitated by the catheter and later, adult diapers. Eleanor saw the humor in my situation and made me laugh whenever frustration undermined my motivation. She also had her own ideas about what would help me get stronger, most notably a concoction of carrots, beets and who knows what else that she made in the blender, and that tasted marginally better than the evil evacuation brew I'd gagged on just prior to surgery. I agreed with her, however, that a vitamin-rich drink would give me strength, so down it went. Eleanor was also a bit of a taskmaster, making sure I did not overextend myself physically. She ran all my errands, did my laundry, changed the sheets, did everything that needed to be done.

Before the surgery, Eleanor and I had not been that close. She mixed with a younger crowd, but she and I crossed paths frequently anyway, often at coffee shops. We'd met through a mutual friend, Eliot "Kidd" Cohen, who had died a year to the day before I had surgery, from a hospital-borne infection following a liver transplant. Eliot had, in his words, "stayed too long at the party" and contracted a terminal case of hepatitis C. I had stayed too long at the party as well, but had never used a needle. I miss both Eliot and Eleanor, who moved away from L.A. after a brief acting stint.

Eleanor was a stand-in of sorts, in that I had expected that other female friend, closer to me, to manage matters after Debbie's return to the Big Apple. But when the reality of my situation hit her, that friend was too upset about the idea of cancer to help me. She expressed some death anxiety about my future, which aggravated fears she had been carrying around all her life. I have since forgiven that fine lady for disappearing on me, but I was quite disappointed at the time. Cancer sure can bring out squirrelly behavior in people.

Not to put her on too high a pedestal or anything, which is a bad tendency of mine, but Eleanor helped in other ways as well. One day she was driving me around Hollywood and I confessed my fears about sex. How would my partner respond to my altered equipment? Would she be freaked out by my dry orgasms and other aspects of the change, which might lead to awkward moments, a more general discomfort and subsequent bigger problems? If we broke up, where would I find a smart, healthy woman who would put up with my beleaguered equipment? Read into that question what you will.

Eleanor had a peculiar answer that covered the possibility that I might find myself back in date mode if Debbie and I could not make it work. "I'm sure a lot of women would find less messy sex quite appealing." Bless her for saying that, as I was having trouble finding the good side to the prospect of handicapped sex, which is how I thought of it in those first weeks after surgery. My male friends had been making jokes about popsicle stick splints and other such ad hoc aids to fulfillment. Rulers at a minimum, please.

As for jokes, let's not discount the transition from catheter to diapers. Once you've healed up enough inside to have the catheter pulled out, you move into diaper mode, which has its own set of psychological issues. Again, for some weeks after the catheter is removed, one simply goes in the diaper without any control, but like almost anything else in life, you get used to it, sort of. Admittedly, driving while your leg is getting warm from the urine pouring out of you can be a bit unsettling, but if you keep an overarching attitude of gratitude about this detour in your life, you should be okay. In the first few weeks of diaper use, expect to change them several times a day, or as often as you expect to urinate. If you drink lots of water, you'll go more often, but water is almost always good for you.

After the ulcer incident, I had put the Vicodin away, relying on acetaminophen for pain, which was not that distracting anymore. It's important to mention that Ibuprofen is a no-no for ulcers, too. Stepping outside myself a bit, I was very curious about how it would feel once a fair amount of testosterone accumulated in my body. Every man knows this feeling well, when sex moves to the front of the mind and stays there until sexual release. I began to feel faint stirrings in the groin, even though weeks had passed since my last climax. My mind had reflexively sublimated the matter for me, allowing me to heal with fewer distractions.

At this point I resolved to recommence the time-honored practice of masturbation forthwith. Whenever archeologists find cave paintings, I am always surprised there are no drawings of a guy pulling on himself. Thankfully, I am not one of those poor souls who finds anything taboo about the activity. I long ago understood that masturbation is akin to breathing and eating, although one should pick one's spots for the former activity with prudence. A man needs to climax when the urge strikes, and in order to regain a feeling of balance, masturbation has sufficed for eons in lieu of a sexual partner, religious and cultural warnings notwithstanding. What's so bad about hairy palms, anyway? Palm clippers, the perfect stocking stuffer.

At the end of the day, Eleanor went home, or perhaps to a coffee shop to think and inspire sweet madness in the minds of men. In my quiet moments, lying in bed in the dark, I monitored how my body was recovering. Hard to tell. Too slowly, for sure. For some reason, while most men find incontinence more distressing than the sexual aspects of recovery, it did not disturb me that much. I was far more worried about getting an erection, maintaining it, and deploying it.

Debbie and I would speak on the phone at least once a day. She made oblique inquiries into how I was feeling sexually, which I brushed off with a few poorly chosen jokes. Looking back, this joking around was a good way to deflect my fears. Call this the wet noodle phase. There was nothing going on in my pants, and I mean nothing in the way of erections. Playing with myself, I grappled with a kind of "What's the point?" depression.

With urgings from both Debbie and Dr. Kuyt to "be patient," I resolved to let things unfold on Mother Nature's healing schedule. But I knew that, for me, to quote a fellow writer who chose to write anonymously in this instance, "patience is the mildest form of despair." The popsicle stick—pardon me, ruler splint—solution was beginning to look viable when to the rescue came my local TV weather girl, Jillian Barberie, a then 30-something hottie who really pushes my buttons. She is married and has a national TV presence now, but back then, only L.A. viewers got to enjoy her wacky, sexy weather reports, as well as her style, fashion, and dog rescue stories. I fit into the latter category, certainly. She can come over and rescue this dog anytime. The salve I needed to rub into my ugly incision scar would have felt good dispensed from Ms. Barberie's fingers. Debbie knows me well enough to know that my fantasies cannot be curbed, so she wisely doesn't try. I'm one of those people who does what he's going to do no matter what, but so far Debbie has been my go-to girl. After all, I love her and I'm glad she puts up with me.

Still, one morning, as an experiment, I imagined myself with Ms. Barberie, who was wearing a nurse's outfit. My fantasy was basically that, in her role as a nurse, her mandate was to help me recover sexually. I recall imagining her sitting on my bed, manipulating me while whispering dirty little nothings in my ear. After a few tries at this tawdry activity, I had a concussive orgasm accompanied by a fountain of urine. Despite the need to change the sheets yet again, it felt great to finally bust out of the patient persona for a moment and to reflect, with a gasp of relief, on the fact that the inguinal nerves were still connected. Somewhat disturbing was the ragged, powerful nature of the climax, as if nerves in my head had short-circuited, causing unnatural sparks to ratchet up my spine and ricochet around in my skull. But I wasn't complaining. I was simply shocked that the nature of orgasm could change along with everything else.

(The bizarre fountain of urine was unexpected and, years later, it still occurs, although to a much lesser degree. This is a rare side effect, so I don't want to harp on it too much, because few readers will experience it.)

I called Debbie at her Manhattan office to share my milestone. She was both giggly and supportive. I cleaned myself up, anticipating Eleanor's arrival. She bounced in with two armloads of groceries and helped me change the sheets. She wondered what had happened, but I did not report my *petit mort,* as the French so quaintly refer to the event. Not surprisingly, I was very much calmer that day, as most men are following sex in the morning. Privately I thanked Jillian B. as she reported on L.A.'s fall weather, such as it is, and I switched the channel to a bad movie that would put me back to sleep. I napped for hours and, when I awoke, Eleanor was still there milling about, having cleaned the apartment. She made lunch, too, which I ate ravenously. Maybe I would be all right after all.

With images of Ms. Barberie dancing, sometimes literally, in my head, working the wet noodle with the fervor of a wayward teenager became my pastime. The key to drier orgasms was to empty my bladder thoroughly just before a "session." It certainly is odd having orgasms without ejaculate and it took me a year before I got acclimated. Perhaps more strange is that the same sensations that propelled sexual activity and release still worked after surgery, although I developed quite a fascination with women's healing behavior. Nurse imagery worked very well up until about 2002, when those mental pictures dissolved as a fantasy resource.

Over the course of the first two months after surgery, the black stitches above my groin gradually dissolved as well. Every morning I would pull some stitching remnants out and wash the "wound" in the shower. Once entirely shaved for surgery, my pubic hair had grown back in and the area would itch greatly by the end of the day. Sometimes I would shower again before bed to keep the itching at bay. Rubbing moisturizer on the healing gash helped also.

As for Jillian B., I just kept thinking of her and, like the little engine that could, my engine could too, a little better each month. Barberie, since married (did I mention that already?) to some guy who I hope appreciates her as the life source she is, embodies both teenager and grown woman. Depending on what mood she's in, she dresses accordingly on camera. At the time of my recovery, I processed her dual nature as a very pleasant, ongoing argument between the immature and more mature elements of her psyche. These observations turned me on very effectively. Some days I could climax twice, though with spacing of 12 hours or more. Steely lightning storms continued in my head during orgasm, although these too abated over time.

Just as the year 2000 approached, I was beginning to believe I would be okay on the most basic level, although I still had very few erections, just a twitch here and there. I had, however, started to regain control of urination. (Word monsters: The act of "making water" is also known as micturition.) Still, there were leaking accidents, sometimes when I drove, as I might not make it to a gas station bathroom in time. I took to driving around with a huge plastic cup in the car, just in case. I think I used it a half dozen times over the first post-op year. You become preoccupied with what's going on with your bladder, and adjust routes and schedules accordingly. A few times at night, I just pulled over on the freeway and urinated behind an open car door, hidden somewhat from the flow of traffic. Motorists could guess what I was doing, but with an urge that strong and uncontrollable, I didn't care what they thought. Had a cop stopped to arrest me, I'd have dealt with that problem in a straightforward fashion. It would have been an interesting ticket to defend in court, but my luck held out and no police intervened.

Work loomed again, as it does for most of us after a medical ordeal. With blood loss from the ulcer escapade, I was slow getting back to it, fatigued and listless. At the time, one of my main employers was one of those zero-empathy types I find both loathsome and fascinating. Once I told him I was ready to return to the keyboard, he loaded me up with some easy work, the key to which is to spread it out over time so the client doesn't think the answers come too easily. This approach dovetailed nicely with my half-broken state, and my output averaged about half of what I usually produced as a business writer on assignment.

An obvious fringe benefit of work was that it took my mind off the angry purple scar that remained after the stitches had fully dissolved. Work also distracted me from the fact that in the first months of recovery I had about five percent of the erectile ability I had had before surgery. I was anxious. As my income had dropped precipitously, I turned to friends for help. Debbie helped tremendously, and one wealthy buddy of mine came through with enough cash to cover months of expenses. I will be forever grateful that he stepped up like that. In return I owe him a TV script, which he has chosen not to collect. He has also helped me in other ways over the ensuing years, but has become a bit elusive recently as his career traverses a distinctive arc.

There is a fine saying in A.A. as one becomes more sober and cogent over the years. "The road becomes narrower." This truism can be interpreted in a number of ways, but I take it to mean that you can't fool yourself once the seriousness of life takes hold. This is not to say that humor isn't one of the more cleansing agents for the soul, but when one recovers from cancer surgery one should quickly learn not to sweat the small stuff. Erections, however, I did not consider small stuff. Insert microscope joke here. You should know that my editor nixed the title *Ups and Downs* for this book, so from the beginning my tendency to make jokes has been under scrutiny, going back to when I rearranged the pots and tops as a kid.

Five

UP AND AROUND

Almost any way you consider it, the prostate gland is odd, and when it comes to surgery, it is about as inaccessible as any human body part. Its main function is to manufacture semen, to perpetuate the species. But like the coccyx (tailbone), it seems to me to be an evolutionary throwback. Evolution has its detractors certainly, most of them thinkers born of, to quote Woody Allen again, "the black hole of imbecility," but it is the weird leftover parts of us that offer perhaps the best evidence that we are descended from lesser, albeit less troubled, creatures. The prostate, like a dense, walnut-sized muscle surrounding the urethra, is taken for granted when we are young. It spasms when properly motivated, and semen erupts accordingly. As we age, we might suffer benign prostatic hyperplasia (BPH), an annoying condition that can enlarge the gland and curtail urine flow. Yet prostate cancer is deadly and common, as it will be the cause of death of about three percent of American men, and it often is less painful or annoying than BPH. It is the disease's "silent" nature that will keep deaths from the disease in five figures annually.

The first radical prostatectomy was performed at Johns Hopkins University in 1904. It was a crude, bleak procedure back then, guaranteeing lifelong impotence if one survived heavy blood loss or infection. Such was a prostate cancer surgery patient's outlook until 1982, when Dr. Patrick Walsh, also at Johns Hopkins, introduced his double breakthrough, low blood loss and erectile nerve-sparing surgery. His first patient, a retired professor named Robert Hastings, was still with us as of the summer of 2007. Pioneer Dr. Walsh has performed upwards of 4,000 such procedures in the last 25 years.

Walsh mapped the complex system of veins and arteries that surround the prostate gland and thereby figured a way to keep blood loss low during surgery.

For nearly 80 years before this, patients undergoing prostate surgery would bleed so much they might die on the table from blood loss alone. Walsh's procedure reduced the mortality rate by 90 percent. From my often nihilistic point of view, death is a zero sum game for the participant, but impotence brings a special negativity to life that I am quite certain I could not manage well. Forty years of depression is enough to overload anybody.

How did couples cope with that sudden reality prior to Walsh's advances? I can barely think about it. Certainly, women in love are the most compassionate, generous creatures on earth, but still, who could blame a healthy woman for leaving her guy if he can no longer fulfill her in that most basic of ways? I suspect this would be more a matter of men's concern than women's, but tell that to the guy whose wife leaves him after the procedure. After all, sex is what draws men and women together initially, so remove that foundation and what is one left with? Perhaps a mad scramble to assess what is left in the relationship, but enough to buttress a future? One would hope that members of long-term couples know each other well enough to embark on the surgical journey as a team or at least to discuss it at length. If you are the man in this equation, do not assume that your wife or girlfriend, especially if she's under 50, will stick around to adapt to your reduced physical circumstances. Talk about it, much as it may be against your nature to do so, or don't be surprised if she leaves. This is harsh perhaps, but we are talking about human beings here, with fragile psyches and the specter of old age whispering in their ears.

Dr. Kuyt's expertise is derived from Dr. Walsh's procedure, and so today I enjoy firm erections when I want them and, unlike in my teen years, never when I do not. But this did not happen in the short term so if, like me, you are impatient by nature, please read closely for some mental tricks I used to get through those long days when I was waiting for a welcome protuberance to enliven those Hallmark moments.

I have alluded earlier to the chronic depression that I suffered from for some 40 years. I have no doubt that it contributed to the uneven road I traveled in recovery. Men who are happy and optimistic by nature will, I am sure, spring back in less time and with fewer emotional hurdles than I faced. Plus, losing pints of blood from the ulcer slowed me down more than the surgery. That said, prior to surgery I had worked hard to integrate my personality, with mixed success. I am still a bit dour some of the time, largely due to years of negative imprinting when I was young.

So by the time my surgery date rolled around, I was still of three overlapping parts, as I recall my frame of mind:

1) My sexuality was largely a separate entity that overwhelmed me on a near-daily basis. Perhaps my testosterone levels were abnormally high, I don't know, but the urge to climax could be crippling at times, since my creative and spiritual selves stood no chance of primacy when I was hotwired for a woman.

2) My spiritual self had been under construction in earnest since December 1984, when I went into rehab and learned about the principles of Alcoholics Anonymous. I had made much progress as a person who made friends more readily and found it easier and easier to uphold his part of the social contract.
3) My creative self was finally beginning to burgeon, as I branched out from writing business articles to screenplays and books. Still, at age 46, I was a long way from being made whole by life's processes, both within and outside my control.

Once the painkillers wore off a few weeks after surgery and I took to tracking my emotional state, I found that my personality had been all but fractured again, just as it had been when my parents' violent acting out dominated my home life, beginning when I was seven years old. Grateful that I was alive and ostensibly in one piece, I also felt as if there were three distinct versions of me: a guy who wrote, a guy who was broken below the belt, and a guy who was piecemeal spiritually. So the challenge in the first few months was not to succumb to feelings that reminded me of being powerless as a kid, powerless in the face of forces much greater than myself. The time to heal that I had mapped out with Dr. Kuyt's help seemed like a prison term: I longed more than anything to get back on the track of self-improvement that I had been on, depression not withstanding.

However, people who suffer from long-term depression discover or create many mental tricks to circumvent both self-pity and self-abnegation. With so little physical energy in those first few post-op months, I could barely make my way around my apartment without having to take a break after 10 minutes. Daily doses of iron pills helped get my blood-making facilities going. I recall one afternoon in particular when I was able to make it to the grocery store on foot, and back, all inside of three hours. This journey should have taken 45 minutes. I got a thorough sense of what it must be like to be 90 years old, and so I no longer get impatient with oldsters who take a long time crossing the street.

As my masturbatory experiments continued along the aforementioned wet noodle track, though featuring ever less urine, I could feel the rat-stem of my brain screaming familiar invectives of self-hatred: "You're a poor, limp, SOB of no use to anyone!" and similar phrases to that effect. Still, my female friends assured me that women don't just drop their guys when such trouble comes along, yet it was difficult to believe them. One may infer that for most of my adult life I had used sex as a drug, to get high rather than close to someone, and for the most part one would be right, although I did learn genuine intimacy along the way.

Funny how the brain works . . . or doesn't. I had to be reminded recently that after the operation the scrotum fills with fluid for the first few weeks after the procedure. Shades of elephantiasis, obvious at the time, but I'd forgotten about it since. It's yet another reason why it's recommended that patients not drive a vehicle, or even a golf ball, during the first few weeks after surgery. Sitting on a sensitive softball-sized scrotum has nothing to recommend it, yet I took to driving a stick shift car too early in recovery. Call me uncomfortable, stupid and mobile rather than safe, prudent and stuck at home, Quasimodo was my mode. Mega-scrotum be damned, my urge to get up and get around town was too great. For me, a restless gearhead who does his best thinking behind the wheel, driving equals living, on some level. Someday, when I am indeed old, someone will take my driver's license away and I will then become the crusty, snarling crank the world deserves, but until then, I will drive. It hardly mattered that I had a urine bag strapped to my leg. Sitting around my place reading grew tiresome quickly. Cabin fever had set in. I had to get out.

Driving, for this Angelino, was a normal activity, psychologically necessary, a way to prove to myself that I wasn't letting slip the oft-referred-to mortal coil. While I cannot speak for lunatic driving cultures elsewhere, in L.A. driving manifests the human life form like nowhere else in the United States. There are buses and a subway system here, which makes sense to some people, but not to me. Buses are a last resort before walking across a county larger than the State of Rhode Island. It just isn't done unless one is disenfranchised or afflicted with the inability to drive. Back then I had yet to join the cell phone brigades, so I had hands enough for driving. Still, it was unwise to get behind the wheel sooner than Dr. Kuyt recommended. With hindsight, I wonder whether it contributed to my urinary problems during sex.

But once my ulcer crisis had passed, I was zooming around like everyone else. Relief slowly replaced gratitude and I began to feel optimistic and even a bit smug. Not a great direction to go in, but off I went. Someday someone will create a sitcom about Angelinos who don't drive. Surely there are couples who hold hands on the buses of L.A. I'd watch that show, in fact.

Returning to the streets of Hollywood meant exposure to the fauna that play there. I visited the Beechwood Café, a restaurant I had frequented, where the waitresses knew about my cancer ordeal. After hugs all around, I sat at the counter next to a young woman who was cute, but with that hardened look of "Don't play games with me, buster!" Just my type. She smiled at me a bit and we exchanged a few mundane remarks about laundry and whatnot. With little motivation to flirt, given I had no ammo in the holster let alone a hard gun, as it were, I kept my place conversationally. That was my first real face-to-face, stranger-oriented, post-op experience of feeling completely disempowered sexually. Rattled, I ate half of my usual portion and went out to my car, feeling hollow. Had I had something witty to say to the woman, I'm not sure I'd have tried that tactic, but as it was, I was shut down and had nothing to say. Once again, it was time to take stock of the positives if I was going to endure the coming months. I needed to dial back from my center-of-the-universe mentality and regain a healthy perspective based on humility.

Some weeks after my encounter with the woman at my favorite lunch spot, I ran into an actress friend who was unaware of my recent life detour. She was tanned, tall, and responsible for global warming. "What's up with you?" she opened with, as I caught myself feeling more dour than usual.

"Prostate cancer. I had it cut out."

"Is that good?" she asked, startled, and I don't recall what I said to her until I blurted out something along the lines of "Do you have a minute?"

I didn't know this foxy lady very well, which suited my purpose. I bought her a burger, over which I regaled her with some feelings I thought I might never get out of my system. She kept her cool as I threw one fear at her after another: I'll never get it up again, what woman will want me? Blah, blah, blah, a litany of self-pity. She was nice about it, as women can be, smiling all the time while she said "Give it time, give it time," over and over again. Then I apologized and left her with money for the bill.

After outings such as these I would go home to reboot my head with a nap, which has always been my routine. I would work a little, rest some more, call my lady in New York City. By the time the evening news came on, I had settled my head enough to regain some self-acceptance, although self-recrimination was always lurking close by. After a couple of months of this routine, I got fed up and made a decision to be more proactive about both socializing and being active physically. And then one morning, Eureka! there came a hint of the familiar engorgement that leads to so many of life's pleasures and problems.

Six

FRUSTRATION, PROGRESS, AND PERSONAL REFLECTIONS

Many writers, and I'm among them, have trouble concentrating on one project at a time. I'm already thinking about another book I want to write, about how American men cope when their primary career plans and vocational dreams don't come true. Some turn inward and spend their time tinkering in the garage. Others shoot up office buildings. Of course this idea has much bearing on this book, too, because frustration is at the core of both ideas. Unless a man enjoys an unusually supportive relationship, he will quietly fend for himself when he realizes that he will never run the company he's toiled at for 20 years, open his own restaurant, or pitch for the Dodgers. The practical requirements of daily life get in the way of the big dreams, as does the matter of insufficient talent, brains, or training. Similar to the guy who comes to this realization about his career is the man who must accept his fate as a diminished sexual being. To the American male, admitting "I can't do it" is one of the most foreign modes of thinking. Is knowing one's limitations a requirement for happiness? I'm not sure—still working on it.

What happens to such men? Some go berserk at times when their dreams are thwarted, hence the term "postal." Men kill their wives and co-workers every day in this country that venerates guns as common household appliances. And women don't get off any easier. They must acknowledge aging as an inescapable offset to wisdom. I knew a woman writer who was sober for 20 years. I had dinner with her and another woman in recovery one Monday night, and shortly thereafter learned that the writer had committed suicide. At dinner we'd been discussing what it meant to lose one's physical attractiveness in the dating world as one got older. This woman could not accept her diminished appeal, and declared that if she couldn't attract a man there was no point in living. I thought she was given to the hyperbole writers are heir to, but no, she soon drank a bottle of vodka and knelt down in the path of an express train. I embrace the creative distinction—a local train would not do. This was the most effective statement of self-annihilation she could think of, to be run over by an enormous metal penis. Was she overloaded with culturally driven imperatives to perform as a sexual being in the American dating marketplace? Absolutely. Every communication medium is awash in sexual imagery tailored to induce anxiety and self-loathing, as typical women are constantly compared to "models" of the female form, six-foot, 125-pound specimens such as Adriana Lima, a Brazilian supermodel who, at 28, is set to lose her virginity on her honeymoon in the summer of 2009. Don't get me started. She lives in a parallel universe. Clothing and accessory designers induce powerful feelings of covetousness to promote what thought designer Karl Marx called "commodity fetishism." Rare is the woman in America or Europe who is immune to it, as sexual power and prowess are the underlying drivers of much of the world's economy. Thus, in America, we come to believe that others see us as the sum of two parts: our jobs and our sex appeal. The market for spirituality is as yet nonexistent, unless one counts organized religion, which I do not.

So, if asked what I am, I say reflexively, "I'm a writer." This identity is so ingrained in me I can't imagine answering any other way, although I am fully capable as a business consultant, and in other roles as well. As for sexual prowess, well, once the initial shock of the surgery wore off, my mind calmed down enough to face the consequences of getting rid of the cancer. In one day, I went from what felt like priapic superhero to a wizened eunuch, or so my personal equipment suggested to me. Adding insult to ignominy was the fact that my pubic area had been shaved for surgery. The bald eagle look was not conducive to romance any more than was a limp penis prone to emitting urine at the most inopportune moments.

Topical hydrocortisone comes in handy when your pubic area has been shaved and the hair is growing back with a maddening itch. I must have gone through a tube of the cream every two weeks until the groin took on a more normal look. The itching was not sufficient to distract me from the humiliating bigger picture, which entailed the absence of hydraulic activity in my boxer shorts. There's nothing like the feeling of walking the streets of a major city when you cannot get it up. Call it a numbing neutrality. Only then does one realize just how much one's personality relies on the potentiality in one's pants. Too much, in my case. The spontaneous flirting I used to be so adept at? Gone. Meeting and holding the gaze of a pretty woman? Gone. With nothing of erectile substance to back me, I now shunned those circumstances. With ladies I already knew, sheepish humor was the best I could muster. Looking back on this especially shaky period, I attribute this temporary shyness to a lingering state of shock, and not to an inherent lack of self-confidence. Had it been the latter, given my depressive tendencies, I would have shut down completely. Instead, I did venture out and about most days.

This severe curtailment of my inner life may sound drastic to most readers not afflicted with chronic depression or bleeding ulcers. Or cancer. Certainly, over the ensuing years I have gotten to know several men who bounced back from RPs rather quickly, with almost no side effects that they would admit to in casual conversation. However, virtually all of these guys acquired a quieter aspect to their personalities, which I surmise may reflect turmoil they either cannot or will not describe. Consider yourself doubly lucky if you do not suffer multiple complications, related or seemingly unrelated to surgery. If you are a depressive person going into the procedure, expect a more irregular recovery, laden with neuroses that you may have been adept at suppressing previously. My point is that major surgery splits you open in more ways than one.

And of course, if your cancer is not caught early enough to remove it all, you are in for a longer haul than I was, with the prospect of radiation and/or hormone therapy, either of which can be very debilitating. Still, what choice do we have? Every man has been faced with forks in the road, both vocationally and in their personal lives. Either you move forward toward some goal and a measure of fulfillment, or you veer off toward limp resignation. Fortunately for me, I have long been fascinated by these philosophical questions and thus I am comfortable when presented with them in real time. This may explain why I got sober the first time I tried to clean myself up. I decided to live, rather than continue to drink and die. It was a clear choice that I made and, after cancer surgery, I was likewise presented with recurring either/or circumstances. I cannot say that I made the most life-affirming choice each time, but on the major questions, I feel I met the challenges effectively because of a preexisting mindset skewed toward gathering thorough self-knowledge. Likewise, in my career, I made a choice in 1989 to be self-employed and I have maintained that status, as I often don't play well with others. Plus, I don't want anyone to take away my propensity to work and watch Gwen Stefani videos at the same time. I want to be watching her *Cool* video on my deathbed.

Which in turn points me to yet another issue. Many men never get to know themselves. Here, in and around Hollywood, it is common to find men stuck in adolescence, as there is no motivation toward maturity as long as the money rolls in. Moreover, the entertainment industry feeds off and condones bad behavior. You may recall the instance of film exec Michael DeLuca, who was widely reported to have been administered fellatio by a girl at a high-profile Christmas party—not in a bedroom but in open view of many guests. Although he was canned by his employer at the time, he was soon hired by a competing company and continues to work in the upper echelons in the industry. In Hollywood, if you have fame and fortune, you might get away with anything, even murder.

Such behavior is indicative of a general trend. Martha Stewart, take note. Is there anyone who believes record producer Phil Spector didn't shoot that blonde actress in the face because she said no? I don't know anyone who doesn't believe it, and yet his first trial ended with a hung jury. I believe these instances to be judicial mutations born of capitalism, and I believe they will continue to proliferate. It will be interesting to see how bad the situation becomes before the American people do something about it.

But back to the effect of personality on recovery. Those of you who have done little soul-searching over the years, do not be surprised when psychological issues come to a head after surgery. No need to list the many possibilities here, as they are as myriad and varied as men are. For many of you, it won't be pretty. Spare your loved ones the worst of it, if you can. It's the big, tough, uneducated guys I worry about the most, the ones wholly vested in a macho persona they have been hanging on proud erections for decades. You know who you are.

Dr. Fred's endorsement of me as the whole man I would again become proved sufficient to get me over the humps, or nonhumps, as the case was, that I faced in those early months of recovery. Fred has so much inherent credibility as both doctor and man that I never questioned his authority on the subject of my recovery.

It should be noted that until the advent of sulfa drugs in the 1930s and penicillin in the 1950s, a doctor's role was historically pastoral, because there was nothing that could be done about many human ailments. Today, a medical doctor's primary role is diagnostic, a great leap forward in some respects, but it also means that many doctors have lost or never possessed that caring, pastoral side. Dr. Fred is an exception.

At his urging, I briefly looked into support groups in L.A. that consisted solely of men who had overcome or were continuing to battle prostate cancer. Then I realized I would not be much of a contributor to such meetings, because my active participation in A.A. served to get in the way of seeking out help in this other area. I had not yet learned that it was fine to sit in a room full of men who were farther along in the recovery process and not say anything. This was odd, because I'm usually a good listener. I don't know how to characterize this mental block, whether it was pride or fear, perhaps both, perhaps something else. If I look deeply enough, I may at some point admit to myself that failure to seek group support in the winter of 1999–2000 was a manifestation of para-suicidal behavior. This reflects the self-destructive streak that runs deep and wide through me, and I know it to be carved out by the part of my mind that wants to capitulate to every self-destructive impulse. This includes acts of omission when I choose not to help myself.

This topic points me to another, larger issue. When you are looking beyond surgery to the recovery process, it's a great idea to choose a plan of support action and stick to it. Learn to take contrary action, behavior I learned in A.A. You may not feel like working out, for example, but you do it anyway because you know the benefits are so good for you. Same thing when helping yourself in other ways. If you're gregarious and outgoing by nature, you're likely to have an easier time of it than the guy who's prone to isolation. I was very good at staring at the ceiling for the first six months or so following surgery. I'm not recommending one go against one's personality when it comes to post-op behavior, because I know better. Is every guy who gets prostate cancer entrenched in his ways? Perhaps all but a few. The stolid introvert is not going to line up outside the local Moose lodge to attend a cancer survivors meeting, but he needs to do something to bolster himself. As a reluctant ambivert, I vacillated between sullen isolation and speaking forthrightly to fellow members of A.A. about my cancer-related issues. I also befriended a wonderful woman named Kay, who has been battling cancer for years. She has been very, very kind to me, and her smile and words of encouragement have gotten me through some tough moments.

To return to my state of mind at the time, other men might have kept their swagger intact, but not me, yet I acknowledge that a man's ego needs to express itself. I slunk around town, ghostlike, running errands, attending A.A. meetings and renting videos. My patience was tested on an hourly basis as I grumbled, staring out the window, wondering how I could improve my energy level and work situation. This angst has its roots in my distrust of authority figures. Like most men who grow up hating authority, respect for my elders was drummed out of me by my father, whose violent alcoholic bent, combined with his unrealized dreams as an actor, taught me very bad lessons.

So when Fred Kuyt, one of the nicest, most sincere men in the world, told me that in time I would be made whole, my inner self heard "You'll live, but you'll be a sexual cripple." Pathetic? Perhaps, but I don't mind expressing my failings, not anymore. I imagine such negativity is difficult to explain to someone who grew up in safe and warm circumstances.

So at the heart of my story is my discomfort over having to deal with authority figures much of the time. It is one of the reasons I treat young people as people, not as incomplete creatures to be condescended to or verbally abused. As a way of healing myself of my hatred of authority, I have learned to trust a few people over the years, but most importantly, I have learned to trust my judgment.

American men are taught, though not in so many words, that leading a meaningful life means largely ignoring one's feelings and staying on a straight, goal-oriented path, if one is physically and mentally able. Young boys see their fathers trudging off to jobs they may hate, sacrificing peace of mind during the day so that they can enjoy their families and their hobbies at night and on weekends. In such families, it is the wife who measures the husband's mood and acts accordingly, either toward improving the family system or dismantling it. This is done consciously and unconsciously, and what goes on in the bedroom is the barometer of the family dynamic. I have seen scores of marriages either develop and flourish or transform into something toxic. How many marriages have you seen that are held together by mere physical attraction, and yet they seem to work? The doctor marries the plumber and, blissful as they are, if they were of the same gender they would rarely cross paths, let alone sleep together. Sex is the weird glue used to cohere disparate personalities as often as congruent ones.

Back in Hollywood, I felt like a has-been porn star put out to pasture, or an extra in an Ingmar Bergman film, emptiness pervading my stance and conversation. My demons, ever a cadre of self-mockery, had a field day. Whereas I typically enjoy assessing a girl's primary asset and making a flirtatious remark about it (them?), if only to generate a bit of repartee, I was at this point brooding in coffee lines and in my walks along Franklin Avenue, where the tattooed and the buffaloed roam, and the queers and the anti-dopers play. I suppressed the urge to call Fred and whine a bit about my floppy penis, and though I knew he would permit some kvetching, I had been trained to shut up and soldier on quietly. This attitude had almost gotten me killed a few times, via bleeding ulcers, but there you have it. I suspect most men are the same way. I recall one of the finest men I have ever known, Mike K., who died in his sleep from the exhaustion of trying to keep his restaurant going. He was around 50 and left a wife and kids. I worry about becoming one of those guys who pushes the Sisyphean rock all his life only to keel over with his boots on.

Perhaps the horrors endured by U.S. soldiers during World War II explain some of the taboo against men speaking up about our issues, but whatever it is, it is not healthy to suppress emotions, and sexual repression or lack of functionality provides a full menu of issues. So, yes, I should have called Fred at least a couple times when I was nearly insane from frustration and worry about the future of my male utensils. In a later chapter I will offer the case of one Leonard Dickman, who has his own way of expressing his frustrations. Leonard's spirit is considerably freer than mine.

Not content to submit to idle self-recrimination, I continued to indulge in fantasies fueled by TV weathergirl Jillian B. and other small screen sirens, which served to keep the hormonal waves crashing on a fevered brainpan. Three months post-op, limpness still ruled the day. But at least I could climax with a metallic, clanging effect that was exhausting. I now realize that these fractured orgasms stemmed from the two inguinal nerves having been bruised during surgery, for over the years this effect has gone away, to be replaced by the more familiar, spine-rattling rapture we all welcome.

Henceforth in this book, in dubious deference to Hollywood's four-star movie rating system, my post-op erections, or lack of them, will be reviewed by the four-towel rating system, that is, how many dry cotton bath towels could be arrayed on my aroused penis before the beleaguered organ became overburdened and the towels slipped to the floor. This measurement of erectile strength reflects both optimism and the benefit of hindsight, for back then I couldn't manage more than a pulsing twinge no matter how much blood flow could be diverted to the fun zone. But a twinge was much better than nothing, as I tried to keep in mind the best advice I ever got in the rooms of A.A., which came from adman Mark S., who advised me one night, "Be kind to yourself."

This phrase may sound ridiculous to many who take self-esteem for granted, as they were likely raised in a safe household with consistently loving parents. But to me, the idea of making a decision to be kind to myself came as a thundering, fresh concept of the best kind. Even today, I find the advice difficult to self-administer. However, a most pertinent example is that I took time away from my normally hectic routine to travel to a quiet town in Colorado, where my dear sister Ingrid and her loving family lives, so that I might write some of this book in the peace and quiet of the Backstreet Bagel & Deli in downtown Ouray. When I get back to L.A. there will be cars to buy and sell and scripts to rewrite and films to make and more books to write, but until then I can sit here and be kind to myself by taking the time to tell a story that I hope resonates with others running the recovery gauntlet of post-prostate cancer surgery.

Three or four months along into my post-op sex life, I rated zero towels, which also rated a half measure of free-floating anxiety. I was reminded of the days of early puberty, at 12 or 14, when, overwhelmed by both newfound energy and an obsession with the curves of the female form, my psyche split into two distinct—what is the word—regions? Domains may be a better word, perhaps too grand. One part of me focused on reading and sports and wondering if my parents were going to kill each other in a drunken rage. The other part of me simply could not fathom how strong the urge was to—what is the word?—devour my budding female classmates. My film icons lured me on TV and in movies. Politics aside, do you recall a 26-year-old Jane Fonda in *Cat Ballou* (1965)? At 12, I staggered out of the theatre with the after-image of the red spangled dress she wore burned into my retinas. The blood of the damned seemed to leak from my eyeballs and somehow down my spine to settle in my lower back, where a second heart seemed to spring forth magically, its sole role to pump hormones and molten steel into my genitals. What would I have done to sink my teeth into Cat's peach-colored calves? Sold my soul cheap? Sure, no problem. Two bucks should cover it. Madness! I sought such women to lead me off into a Dantesque world of steaming carnality. Bring on the babes!

Barely recovered from Miss Fonda's turn in that underappreciated comedy Western, I then beheld Gina Lollobrigida in *Hotel Paradiso* (1966). This Italian bombshell, and her equally compelling countrywoman Claudia Cardinale in *The Professionals* (1966), scarred me for life. Even today, a dark Mediterranean woman with mercurial mischief driving her personality can reduce me to salivating stupidity in seconds. I believed Gina knew everything important there was to know. If only Gina lived down the road from me in my somewhat quaint Connecticut hometown! Surely she would have taken a liking to me, comprehended the ocean of urgency that lurked in my shivering testicles and set out to make a man of me by sharing her hidden secrets and endowing me with panty souvenirs. Alas, I was to wait until I was 16 to find a heavenly hiding place for my penis, and in the intervening years, how much of my mental time and energy was focused on the other gender? Fully 70 percent I'm sure, perhaps more.

This reality would have been more manageable had someone warned me about its impact. Polynesians warn their children about the potential of tsunamis, so what was there no warning for me when puberty struck without so much as a heads up from anyone? There are ads in the back of the *New York Times Magazine* for camps for fat kids and kids of various creeds. What about a camp for horny kids? One summer with a bevy of hot 18-year-old female counselors, where there were no fascist cultural stigmas about sex, and I would have gained an understanding of the ebb and flow of natural sexual energy and been straightened out for good. I'm sure such a torrid summer would have spared me 15 years of excessive drinking to try to heal my inner wounds and frustrations, not the least of which stemmed from the eternally vexing question of where to put it.

When I was a senior in high school, I wrote a short story about teen sexual frustration. I received an F for my efforts and my parents were warned about the nature of the child they were raising. I will soon rewrite that story for publication. My father didn't care and my mother knew that my mind had been gouging out a path in the gutter for some years. Back when I was 11, in the middle of watching *Mary Poppins,* I'd been sent out of the theater to wait in the car for the remainder of the film for my very audible, in-theater comment about Julie Andrews' "bazookas." In 1966, two years later, I snuck into the same theater with my friend Paul to see the x-rated *Blow-Up*. Looking as always for extremes, I was disappointed, as my reading material had already gone to darker sexual realms.

In 1967, I gawked at Brigitte Bardot in *And God Created Woman* and wondered if there was a way to construct a life whereby I could have stayed in bed with BB all day and night, every day and night. This arrangement seemed perfectly reasonable then, and it's even more so today. I'm convinced that within this motive is the original initiative for take-out food.

At age 16, rating four towels would have been no problem, even soaking wet (the towels, not me). Readers will recall those days when, as certain rock lyrics intone so gracefully, a cat couldn't scratch it. Or, if I may paraphrase a line from the Catskill comedians, snow lingered on the tip in the summer. And I can still recall the rage I felt at how the culture I lived in was structured. In order to find supple lodging for that most insistent of organs, one was required to adhere to a set of time-honored rules. In a word, dating. What a ridiculous idea. No one told me that girls were wired altogether differently, that courtship allowed the girl to get to know her suitor before she gave up that most tender of prizes. I had assumed that a girl's ideas were her most prized possession, reflecting what I prized in myself, but a few years of close pubescent observations disabused me of that notion. The reality was that one had to find the occasional libertine among girls, the one who came from a broken home or gave it away as a way to get attention.

Where would the world be without those sporty girls? Every high school has them. I suspect there would be a Columbine-type incident every week in this country without those girls who say yes to often loveless propositions. Still, generally speaking, there is no more frustrated creature on earth than the alienated teenage male in America. No one's chain is yanked harder, no one is subject to more temptation. It's something of a miracle that young American guys get through adolescence at all, given that the rules of dating are there to protect girls and prohibit an outlet for boys. I can remember being extremely jealous when a 16-year-old peer's dad drove him into New York City to partake of the services of a hooker, whom the dad paid for. This kid went on to be a hit with the ladies, as he brimmed with the confidence of knowing. Say what you will about the morality of such an initiation, what this country reveres more than anything else is results, and the penis and gonads are a very results-oriented team.

Returning now to my status around three months post-op, despite a zero-towel rating, the good news for me was that the nerve endings were still attached and orgasm was achievable, albeit accompanied by a fountain of urine in my case. But boys will be boys, so I was soon on the phone with Debbie pleading for her to come out from New York for some play time. She was nice about it, loving me and all that, so out she came and played we did. Her role had much of the nurse to it, as the sex was nonvigorous, not something you'd see in an outtake of *9 1/2 Weeks*. Most of the time I worried about urinating in the bed. Debbie understood my frail state and administered the attention that a zero-towel rating warranted. No doubt my academically oriented editor would draw the descriptive line here regarding our nonacademic behavior, so I will draw the line for her.

Resting after a session of clinical, therapeutic sex, it was easier to muster the A.A. aphorism about an "attitude of gratitude" that would make or break my recovery. In A.A., there is a plague of false humility, especially in L.A. I have caught myself acquiring this ugly trait from time to time. so in the last few years I have gone to recovery meetings only sparingly, to remind myself of where I've been and of what awaits me should I go back to drinking. In L.A., what passes for gratitude can often be mistaken for repressed aggression concerning either one's exalted place in the entertainment industry or one's wannabe status. These are the thwarted dreams of those on the inside looking out. With my damaged psyche, exposure to either state of mind was poisonous.

In my A.A. experience, the atmosphere at New York meetings is not this way, reflecting something positive about the much more mature City on the Hudson. By the close of 2008, I'd attended something like 2,000 A.A. meetings, so I'd had plenty of exposure to both the great and the avoidable in that very well-meaning organization. My point is that I am always on the lookout for influences that will either aid in integrating my personality or in disintegrating it. I look favorably on both pursuits, depending on which day you ask me.

Other than our mutual tending to my physical needs, during Debbie's visit I didn't take the opportunity to talk at length with her about how I was feeling, which was on the order of "If I can't get it up again, I will disappear into a cabin in the Alaskan wilderness to write nihilistic stories themed around castration." I would eat venison, I decided, acquire a hardy mutt to hunt with me and stare adoringly at me and call it a day. Instead, I probably offered her nonverbal cues about how I felt, and she dealt with my passive-aggressive tendency to self-embalm with my own gastric juices. Much as I am an advocate of the proven dialectical method for getting at the truth, I am not a great practitioner. Intellectually I know talk is good when you are healing from anything, but my own medicine rarely goes down easy.

Speaking of speaking, I heard that in a recent study of college kids it was reported that young women averaged 16,000 spoken words per day and young men 15,000 per day. The girls' number I get, but who are these guys in the survey, gay students of interior design? Fifteen thousand spoken words might be my monthly output, and I'm sure that at times in some months I have written more than I've spoken. This is a habit with much productivity to recommend it when one is not recovering from major surgery, but given my anxiety level about my erectile future and persistent partial incontinence, I can now recommend to you that, if your prostatectomy number is up, you talk a blue streak to someone about everything that's on your mind. In short, be kind to yourself.

Seven

CONTINENCE AND CAMARADERIE

It is part of the Darwinian equation that some men will die of prostate cancer because they are ignorant, while some take pride in ignorance. It's that simple, and that sad. Back in August 2001, I attended my 30th high school reunion. My article in the *Washington Post* had just been published, and several of my classmates had read it. Reaction was positive, yet some of the men, 48 years old, said they'd never go to the doctor unless they had unbearable pain. I took a few of them aside and explained the medical realities to them, to no avail. Despite their assurances that they would think about having their prostates checked when they turned 50, I could tell they would have to be damned lucky to make it to old age. Dinosaurs come in contemporary forms.

Even more alarming is that there are some men who will avoid the urologist's office because of incontinence or the fear of it. If you have a wife or significant other, the best chance for you to break through the defiance is to hear the advice from her. We all know that the effectiveness of advice is more often dependent on source than content. Please consider that if you are mulling over what to do about your positive diagnosis. Too many guys subscribe to the watchful waiting school only to be told a year down the road that they have an aggressive form of the disease. Better to have the cancer addressed when your PSA is 5 rather than 500.

Let's take a detour here to heed voices of my comrades in treatment. A nagging voice in the back of my mind instructs me to provide readers with other points of view about the main issues in this book. The best way to do that is to reprint some of the e-mails (last names absent) I received in response to the *Washington Post* article. After all, it was these e-mails that prompted this book. I think it is very important for readers of my story to get perspectives from other men who have had prostate cancer. Plus, some women chime in as well. The article was published on August 14, 2001, on the front page of that paper's health section. I realize that my take on recovery may not resonate with some readers, so perhaps the following writings will help sort things out for them. I should caution you that some of the writers had terminal disease. I include the writers' compliments to me not to boost my ego but to show that the points I'd made in the article had hit home.

It is only fitting to begin with the letter penned by the late Robert Vaughn Young, whose response to being diagnosed (November 23, 1999, at age 61, with a PSA of 1,000) was to start a purposeful Web site at www.phoenix5.org. Robert and I corresponded several times over the years. A retired writer, Young chronicled his fight until he passed away on June 15, 2003. The site is still active, and I especially recommend Robert's journal. People say I have courage in writing my story. My story is a piffle compared to his. Robert wrote to me the very morning my article came out. Out of respect for him and his widow, Caren, I repeat his letter here in its entirety, as I'm sure Robert would have wanted:

> *I am (happily) stunned that the* Post *would print such a story. Since such graphic accounts have been reserved primarily for a couple of books, e.g., Michael Korda's* Man to Man, *I can well appreciate their little warning.*

The *Post* had warned their readers that delicate sensibilities might be offended by the truth I was revealing. I declare that some tightly corseted ladies outside the Beltway might've taken the vapors.

> *I was diagnosed with prostate cancer 21 months ago that was too advanced (called "end stage") for any option but hormone therapy, which took away my potency and libido. For the last 18 months, I have devoted myself exclusively to trying to help other men (and their companions) with the effects of the disease, primarily through Phoenix5.org, a web site that I created for this purpose. Thus I have not only my own intimacy with the disease and its effects but through correspondence with literally thousands of men (and women) around the world, I have become quite familiar with the full range of devastation the disease—and the treatments—can create and the lack of support.*
>
> *Such effects—as you fully know—are what prostate cancer (and treatment) is about. It can destroy more than a life. It can destroy a man's dignity, his identity and his feeling of worth and then take the same tragic toll on his relationship and family. I know that part intimately. When I sought help as the effects of my treatment dug into me to the point that I wanted to die, I found that books and even web sites gave but a passing mention to the effect on a man's identity. So I created phoenix5 to help fill that gap, which really taught me how much yet has to be done.*

To now see the issue coming to the fore in a publication like the Post, *gives me hope that men and women will have a chance to openly discuss it even more. As Viktor Frankl said in his* Man's Search for Meaning, *when we are no longer able to change a situation, we are challenged to change ourselves and how we meet it is how we give meaning to our lives. Sadly, too many men cannot do it. They (and their companions) feel alone and they give up. Your story brings some hope and a chance that this can change. I commend you. I commend the* Post *for publishing it. Life is, as you say, good and you just made it better.*

It is very tough for me to retype those words with dry eyes.

A somewhat high-profile professional in the cancer field responded with:

I was diagnosed in January 1999 at age 49 (PSA 8.5, Gleason 7), and after using all the resources at my disposal both in the (organization) and among my friends in the medical community, I also chose surgery . . . I have just last week had my fourth of 10 semi-annual check-ups with a PSA of zero . . . During follow-ups when my doctor asks about sexual function, I have to say "it's like my golf game, inconsistent." You have cited all the factors that can have an impact on making love . . . I had figured to die in my 90s, shot by a jealous husband, as the old joke goes.

Everybody's a wise guy.

A great deal of my identity and self-worth are and were found in my sexual ability. The good news is that most of that creativity and inventiveness is still there even if one anatomical part may not always be. It is really important for survivors like us to talk about this and to demystify the process if we are going to save more lives.

Another respondent, Jerry, on the east coast, had this to add to the mix:

My PSA was 29 when discovered; I had no real alternative except radical prostatectomy in 1992 . . . Went eight years with PSA below 1.0 and then a sudden rise to 6.0. Physicians prescribed Casodex (oral) and injections of Lupron. PSA is once again below 1.0.

Jerry was part of a long-term study of men who had undergone RPs. Fully 30 percent of them had cancer recur within 10 years of surgery, but Jerry does not say if the thousands of men in the study were chosen randomly among RP patients or because their PSAs were high at original diagnosis, as his was. It is worth noting that the men who responded to my *Post* article were overwhelmingly those with PSAs in single digits, which usually signifies that the cancer has not breached the capsule wall. The guys with the very high end-stage scores are conspicuous by their silence, just as I would have been had that been my fate. It is very humbling to consider those guys who are finding their often isolated way.

A guy named Don had a handle on things. An excerpt from his e-mail:

> *While I have never had the disease (age 48), my older brother has. Your article has helped me prepare for its eventuality.*

Right on, Don; that's the genetic ticket.

A guy named Robert mentions the issue that was a big deal for me in the first few years after surgery:

> *Now it's very different. No depression, thanks to Paxil, no real melancholy, but this sense that the ladies are beautiful, delightful, but I'm no longer in play. That's the huge difference . . . One last thing, an old Irish saying. We spend the first 25 years developing a body, the next 25 developing a mind, the next 25 developing a soul. And God bless the cancer survivors who haven't been able to catch it in a jar.*

No Longer in Play, the title of someone else's book, was written by a not-so-mythical guy whose erectile nerves were not spared.

Nils from Finland sent me a long e-mail. He happened to be in Washington, DC, at the time and picked up a copy of the *Post*. I was not pleased to read how his urologist advised him:

> *I'm 56 . . . I went for a routine check-up. My PSA was 4.5 . . . but my physician found a small bump on the left side of my prostate.*

He found a urologist, had a biopsy, and the urologist was ready to operate. Meanwhile he took hormone pills that stifled his libido. He had to use Viagra to keep his girlfriend smiling. Then back to the dubious urologist.

> *Mentally he was up to his elbows in blood . . . After some discussion he said, "OK, if orgasm is that important to you we'll settle for radiation." He had, fairly enough, warned that surgery could damage the nerves.*

Nils concluded by quoting a Finnish proverb: "Life is dangerous—you won't escape it alive." Something is wrong with Nils' picture, but I'm not sure what.

An oncology nurse took the time to write:

I see many prostate cancer patients at the end stage of their lives . . . In reading your article I laughed, cried and empathized. I pray that your words can be an inspiration and motivation to others. Continued good health.

One of the longest notes I received was from Barry, who sent me two pages on August 15, 2001, the day after the article was published. Here are some excerpts:

I too was diagnosed with PC at age 55. Your letter [sic.] is the first I have seen that deals with the lifestyle situations as opposed to medical situations . . . I spent 1½ years looking into my choices of treatment.

Readers, if you have prostate cancer, do not take this long to decide a course of treatment. A month is long enough, as the disease marches on relentlessly.

I interviewed every urologist, radiologist and nuclear medicine doctor in the [HMO] *system. Each had a different spin on treatment. All felt that because of my profile, i.e. age, health, Gleason, etc., that surgery or broad beam radiation was the ticket. Not one doctor ever asked me what I wanted out of treatment, how I viewed PC, death, sex, etc. It was all about a CURE* [his caps], *which is at best only 40% assured.*

I had never heard anything like that poor a percentage number assigned to cancer confined to the prostate. Had Barry's cancer made a break for other parts of his body? Or was it just his nefarious HMO covering its ass?

Barry balked at the knife.

The radiologist reluctantly agreed to do "the kitchen sink" treatment of hormones, broad beam and seeds. Because of the high probability of incontinence, impotence and other damage caused by broad beam my CHOICE [his caps] *was hormones and seeds. I accepted the fact that my choice was not the best choice from a medical standpoint but I felt it was best for my needs and feelings. By the way, I am a bachelor that has been fairly active sexually my adult life and warehoused much of my identity in that sexuality. I attended "man-to-man" meetings, investigated Internet sites, chat groups, and interviewed PC survivors. I had acquired a fairly deep understanding of PC. No one talked about sex, life, feelings, etc. It was always other factors as though quality of life wasn't in the mix. The man to man group always invited wives to participate. That left the discussion at a polite level and very sterile. Upon my request, the wives were uninvited and the "boys" started talking, but still very medical and not much to lifestyle issues. By the way, most of the surgery patients had some long term damage although I will confess that most were in their 60s or older.*

Eventually, Barry found a doctor who would "*talk TO me and not AT me.*"

Larry also gets right to the point. This was his entire e-mail:

As I'm sure you've noticed, candid and straightforward reporting on this topic is virtually nonexistent.

Not anymore, Larry, not anymore.

From the ladies' side of the street I received this from Linda:

Your article was honest and thorough—but remember there is the mental bonding between man and woman—which I believe goes much beyond the physical. It is the sharing of feelings—the open dialogue where men and women fumble—trying to save face . . . it manifests itself in small gestures—hugs, kisses, holding hands, leaning on and lying next to each other . . . it replaces and becomes the sex for your next stage of development . . . few men and women do it well . . . many die without reaching this stage of development.

Okay, lady, sure.

You ended your article with life—which you still have—it's good . . . enjoy it while you can.

A man named Joseph wrote this response, also dated August 15, 2001. This note was very satisfying for me:

I can't believe your experience in this process. I just had my prostate removed 6/21/01 and was on the phone with my MD who sent me to your piece. I was cranking on him as to my "after effects" which are nearly exactly as you state. The good news is it looks like there is actually light at the end of my tunnel and that IS a good thing . . . Finally your comment about "pensive" is dead on with my state of mind but I hoped that it would go away soon. You say this more than two years later?

Yes, I did, in a publication distributed worldwide. As did many respondents to the article. Jim wrote on August 15, 2001, as well:

I am scheduled for surgery August 22, 2001. My surgeon, after two opinions, suggested complete removal. I agreed. He will perform a "nerve-sparing operation" and I should be able to have an erection in the future after my recovery process. I was very much amazed at you mentioning in your article about wearing diapers/Pampers! My doctor has not mentioned anything about me doing what you had to do. I too will have a catheter in my penis for just that purpose . . . My PSA was 4.1 . . . I'm still traumatized by what I'm going through even at this moment. I too have a very sexual life. I am 51 years old and feel like I'm 21 . . . But my life will be changed emotionally and physically . . . Thanks so much for your openness in your article. Right now, I am at a stage of this process where you used to be.

Another guy named Jim wrote to me the very day the article was published:

I read your article with great sympathy. I was diagnosed in 1998 at age 44. PSA 26–30. Gleason 7. Like you, I had no symptoms, and my problem was diagnosed through a stroke of luck. I had a radical prostatectomy in February '99 (no nerve sparing), followed six months later with brachytherapy.

Jim with the RP/brachytherapy one-two punch continued:

Until a few weeks ago, I remained hopeful that these treatments had done the trick with my fairly advanced disease, as my PSAs came back less than 0.1. The last PSA shows a slight rise to 0.2, however, so my wife and I are holding our breaths to see if this is just a fluctuation or the beginning of a steady rise . . . This has been quite a hurdle for me as my surgery did not spare the crucial erection-guiding nerves. I've had to relearn how to have sex, and it hasn't been easy. Everything you mentioned about the lack of spontaneity and the awkwardness—and more—applies.

I wrote to Jim again recently, late in 2008 and received a response. I have edited out Jim's current doctor's name and the school where he taught. This update speaks very loudly about a couple of issues:

Beginning in about 2002, my PSA began to rise again. Happily, I came into contact with an oncologist with whom I've been consulting ever since. He, too, suffers from PC and was treated radiologically. He was forced to leave his faculty position, but has opened his own practice in Virginia, where he treats patients from all over the world. He has a chemistry background and has given great attention to the role of diet and dietary supplements in the treatment of PC. He is also very savvy about the evolving knowledge of the chemistry underlying PC and treats with some radical medicines. The fact that I'm still around (now nearly 55) after my bout with aggressive PC in 1999 is proof that I'm a lucky beneficiary of his cutting-edge theories. My PSA has begun rising again in the last nine months and is now slightly over 10. The rise began when one of the key medicines I was taking, Leukine, was taken off the market by its manufacturer, Baxter. The reason was that it is principally used in treating certain forms of leukemia (not PC) and was causing sudden drops in blood pressure in elderly patients. I will see my doctor again in February, and resuming Leukine is an option now that it's back on the market. Hormone therapy is another possibility, as I may not yet be hormone refractory. He also has some additional chemical cocktails in mind. So I should be around for another few years assuming we can keep the PSA under control.

My biggest complaint these days is urological. I was treated with brachytherapy in August 1999, six months after my unsuccessful radical prostatectomy. This was an unusual course of treatment. The idea was to irradiate the prostatic bed heavily in the hope that the disease had not spread too far afield and might be attackable there. Although the radiation ultimately didn't work, it kept the disease in check long enough for me to find my current doctor. So on balance it seems to have benefited me. Nevertheless, in 2003 I began having incontinence problems. Ironically, I also began having urinary retention. These conditions have now progressed to the point where I'm completely incontinent, except for when I'm completely blocked and unable to urinate. Both conditions are the result of radiation scarring. I had no idea the effects of the brachytherapy would manifest themselves so severely and so many years after the treatment. The urological problems I now face are not remediable, and they are sometimes painful. But they beat the alternative.

Thanks for the update, Jim. Very informative.

A quick note from a woman, Hilary, again the day of publication:

You don't know me from Adam—

Oh, yes, I do, Eve.

—but I just finished reading your article in today's Washington Post *and I had to e-mail you and say BRAVO* [her caps], *and thank you for having the courage to write about your experiences so eloquently and with such sensitivity. I am certain that your words will help many people and inspire many more. Wishing you the best of health always . . .*

Those of you wondering what I got out of this process of revealing my inner life in crisis, this brief note should answer most questions for you. Interesting that there is no mention of a cancer-afflicted man in her life.

Also on publication day, Stan wrote to me:

Your article in the Washington Post *Health Section is outstanding, humanly written and offers great insight into the emerging area of information and awareness about prostate cancer. I am a founder—along with a well-respected urologist—of a highly credentialed urological web site called www.hisandherhealth.com.*

As of late 2008, this site was still very deep with good information and I recommend it highly, though Stan is no longer there.

On a note of bonding, there was this from Allen:

> *Just wanted to congratulate you on your well-written article concerning your prostate surgery published in today's* Washington Post. *Here's wishing you many more years of great performances by that most useful of all body parts. Well done!*

And well put. It gave me a different kind of good feeling to hear from people who expressed no cancer issues.

A man named Claude wrote to me from outside the U.S. on August 13, 2002, more than a year after the article appeared, and six months after he had had an RP. He wanted to know

> *How many months after the operation were you able to have regular sex? I am also taking Viagra and also doing some of the things the doctor advised, but still nothing. I do have an orgasm when oral sex is performed, but my penis is still soft.*

I wrote to Claude a few times and never heard back from him. I tend to experience a little bit of free-floating anxiety when someone establishes contact and then disappears. It's not in my nature to do something like that at all, unless someone's being malicious. Seems to me as if Claude had intimacy issues.

Another guy named Rick, age 60, wrote to me on October 16, 2001. He was to have his RP on October 29, 2001, at his local HMO:

> *Luckily, the HMOs here keep you in the hospital as little as possible so I am going in at 9 A.M. for an 11 A.M. operation, and my wife will be with me. She's ultra-supportive; I'm lucky if they approve a two-day stay.*

I wrote back to him recently at his work e-mail address and the e-mail bounced back. He was probably retired. Rick is lucky his HMO did not have a drive-through OR. That's a skit I should pitch to *Saturday Night Live.*

Then there was Donald, whose September 15, 2001, sounded very emotional. (Note that I choose my tenses carefully, as I am hopeful everyone who wrote to me early in the decade is still alive.):

> *I hope you have been doing better than me . . . I have been feeling a little lonely at times, not being able to function, not being able to live life as I know it. I've also been isolating a little. This is a real trauma for me, period. But I'm progressing. Every day I'm getting better.*

That's the spirit that gets us through this ordeal, I thought. Further along, he wrote:

> *It has been since August 17th that I have been out of work not making a salary . . . For the past 10 years I work in the consulting business where you have to be on contract and being on contract, if you don't work, you don't get paid period. In my industry there is no advance sick leave or employees contributing leave. We have short term disability, but that does not activate until after 90 days. I'm one of those cases that people talk about that falls through the cracks.*

Here was a guy—a good taxpayer, one presumes—living in the world's richest country, still with no universal healthcare. Maybe he'd been wiped out by digging into his savings. We can only hope we get coverage for all U.S. citizens soon. Donald's letter is worth quoting some more, as he found a support group in his area

> *that meets on the third Tuesday of every month . . . Now that the nerve-sparing surgery is over, I have all kinds of fears about my ability/inability to achieve and or maintain an erection. I know I'm probably too much in my head at this point, but I have been reading and reading materials about the potential impact on male sexual health after prostate surgery . . . Please give me your feedback. I'm just an emotional wreck right now. But I know I have to maintain some type of sanity because stress and depression will not help me at this point in time, especially through my healing process.*

A man after my own well-trammeled heart, this Donald. I wrote to him then and my text got through. Donald concluded his missive with, "*I just want to be able to function sexually again soon and not feel that I have a 50/50 chance of NOT* [his caps] *performing.*"

I spoke with Donald on December 22, 2008, and again a few days later. He said he was doing pretty well but recently his PSA had crept up to 0.2, after being negligible since his treatment. His doctor was keeping an eye on him, having him come in for checkups every six months. Donald had never been told what his original Gleason score was, so I made sure he got up to speed and found out that it had been 6.0. Donald had never heard of the Gleason scale until I mentioned it to him.

From the distaff side of the healing equation, I heard from Lucita on August 13, 2002, a year after the article's publication. She wrote,

> *I have a friend who was recently diagnosed with prostate cancer, and is in the process of evaluating the treatment options. He's 44 years old.*

Her friend was leaning toward radiation therapy, and that choice made me wonder how he'd made out. I'm sure I wrote some words of support at the time. Like many of my correspondents, Lucita's e-mail address was no longer valid when I attempted to follow up with her toward the end of 2008. Moreover, I would have liked to know how a 44-year-old discovered he had prostate cancer. Maybe there is some internalized detection method I am unaware of that would certainly bear scrutiny. If you know of something other than an altered urine stream or routine physical that alerted you or someone you know, please write to me at johnhallen borg@aol.com so I can disseminate the information.

Another gentleman, Fred, wrote to me on September 9, 2001, three weeks after my article appeared and two days before the world was forever changed:

> *Thirteen years ago, at age 44, my urologist hit me with a 2 by 4 following a routine biopsy. Through a digital check my family doctor had detected a bump on the shell of the walnut.*

Note: a DRE did not reveal anything in my case as my two tumors were in the interior of the gland. Hence the importance of the DRE and PSA tests cross-checking each other.

> *This was at the end of a physical exam I had requested due to job stress. I felt his insistence to complete the physical with the bendover exam was not necessary since I felt fine in that area, it was my heart I was worried about. He sent me to my urologist who did his own DRE. He said I was too young and too healthy to have a prostate problem, but there was a bump and he wanted to check it out to be sure. From there your article fits me like a glove.*

This idea, that a man who seems to me brimming with health cannot be harboring a death warrant deep in his body, is something that must be eradicated if we are going to have any chance of eradicating prostate cancer itself.

Fred continued:

> *My wife has been my strength. My emotional make-up is stoic on the outside, but inside I have often been a mess. She knows my moods and has been able to guide me thru low periods. I want to thank you for putting into writing what I experienced. It says what I have felt and experienced but have not shared with others. I have shared the article with family and friends. It does what I have been unable to verbalize, even to my wife. Thank you.*

Rather than being flattered, my first reaction was; Why did it take until 2001 for an article like mine to be published? It's very disturbing that such an important topic could be buried for so long. Fred went on to explain that he was cured, yet his feelings about the surgery still lingered.

Which brings me to Wes, whose RP was performed September 1997. He also wrote to me September 9, 2001. I was glad to read that he had seen my article, not in the *Post*, but in the National Prostate Cancer Coalition's e-magazine, which apparently licensed the piece:

> *Since you are a professional writer, one would expect the article to be well written; however, honest candor does not always accompany such writing.*

Ain't that the truth.

> *I've had great difficulty getting people—both lay and docs—to discuss the "leaking problem" as it relates to sexual activity. I had begun to think I represented a rare occurrence re this problem.*

His leakage, like mine, is quite rare, though. Lucky us.

> *Your insight was very helpful to my psyche.*

At the time he wrote to me, Wes told me his PSA was undetectable, but without going into details, he added, "*I have my share of problems from my rendezvous with the disease.*"

Nonetheless, Wes continues to be very active in the fight against PC. A retired healthcare administrator, he works for the Department of Defense's $80 million a year research effort into a cure for PC. You can access the details of this program here: http://cdmrp.army.mil/pcrp/

And this was from Rick, who also wrote to me on September 9, 2001 (it seems the Coalition's e-mag prompted a number of guys to write):

> *I too was diagnosed with prostate cancer in October 1999. I was 51 and my PSA (6.1) sent red flags up that something was going on.*

He missed a chance for a good joke there.

> *I had a radical prostatectomy on December 1, 1999 and what a way to bring in the year 2000. My how life changes with a simple blood test. Hindsight being 20/20, I would do the same thing all over again. I really had no problems with surgery but the doctors failed to tell me about "retention."*

This is when one simply cannot urinate and the bladder needs to be drained with the medical help. Bad cases can lead to uremia, a potentially dangerous condition.

Three times I had to go to emergency for retention. I became less and less afraid of the catheter each time. My urologist told me that I had one tiny spot that came up positive near the bladder. I started radiation treatments in February 2001 and the last one was April 13, 2001, for 37 treatments in all. Radiation I feel is worse than surgery as radiation has a tendency to creep up on you and makes you feel tired.

I'll bet. Thirty-seven freakin' treatments?

I am doing fine now and everything is back to normal except erections. There is always hope. PSA tests have all come back .01 . . . I am a Vietnam veteran (1969-Navy) and the VA has stated that if you were in Vietnam, you were exposed to Agent Orange. Who knows but there is some scientific proof that there is an association with prostate cancer and Agent Orange. The average age for the Vietnam veteran is 54 and the VA expects to see more Agent Orange related diseases. I hear pros and cons about the PSA test but my doctor and the PSA saved my life.

Here's a stand-up veteran suffering from the government's ongoing disinformation campaign to deflect the blame for exposure to chemical agents, brought to us by the very people who shoved our boys down the meat grinder of a half-fought war. Bless the veterans, one and all, as they did fine service.

Checking in from the fairer gender's perspective was Carol, who wrote to me and to the health editor of the *Post* on August 26, 2001. I don't know if she's a doctor, but she corrected me on a couple of medical points.

Mr. Hallenborg lists some options for treating prostate cancer—prostatectomy, radioactive seed implants, hormone therapy, and chemotherapy—but left out one very common, effective treatment—external beam radiation that can now be more accurate with conformal methods of IMRT (intensity modulated radiation therapy, see www.nomos.com).

I mention beam radiation in this book a few times.

He also stated that the prostate gland and the seminal vesicles generate semen. The testicles produce the sperm that are also part of the semen; the prostate and seminal vesicles contribute the fluid that is added to the sperm.

As long as I am able to stand, I am pleased to stand corrected as well. Carol went on to imply that her husband had advanced disease and passed on after some treatment.

Michael from Israel wrote to me on August 26, 2001:

I am aged 54 and underwent a prostatectomy just seven weeks ago. Like you, the fact that I had cancer was revealed following a PSA test. I too remember the scary, bloody ejaculation following the biopsy—something they should have warned us about.

He certainly has a point there.

My wife thought her period had come early! From here on, however, our paths went in different directions. I had read about the use of the laparoscopic, robotic surgical techniques being pioneered in Paris, France and chose to undergo my prostatectomy there. I was in hospital several days and the catheter was removed before I was released. There then followed weeks of weakness and discomfort, particularly when I tried to sit for lengthy periods, but I have been dry since the operation and am not having to wear pads . . . As for erections, it is early days yet and, although I get some swelling, it is far from being a full erection . . . It is important that people know what they are getting themselves in for. However, the alternative to medical treatment is hardly preferable.

LaVonda's husband must have had a tougher go of it. She wrote me on August 24, 2001:

I just finished reading your article in the Post *regarding prostate cancer. At the risk of sounding like a brainless simpleton I'd like to say W*O*W!!!!!!!*

She was excited at the time, but I was hesitant to write to her in late 2008, based on what followed:

My husband was diagnosed in February 1999 with a Gleason of 9/10. We had HDR (high dose rate brachytherapy, radioactive seeds) in September 1999 and are now on intermittent hormone therapy. We're doing quite well in keeping the PSA below undetectable. I'm so glad to hear you are also doing well. Thank you for bringing to light some of the changes that occur when cancer decides to become your houseguest. I like to think of it as the houseguest from hell. Great job, John! It was an EXTRAORDINARY [her caps] *article filled with information that is sure to stir the hearts of many. Dialogue is what is needed to fight the good fight as best we can.*

I did write to her on December 16, 2008, but with her husband's very high initial Gleason score, I dreaded her response. Alas, her e-mail bounced back to me. Further research produced her phone number, so I called her. Her husband Charlie is doing great. Although his cancer had escaped to the seminal vesicles, his doctor has placed the temporary radioactive seeds there. Also, he had beam radiation as a follow up. LaVonda said his PSA, which was 6 or 7 at diagnosis, was now negligible. With a Gleason of 9/10, that's a fortunate outcome indeed.

I received this e-mail from Stephen on August 23, 2001:

My cousin had forwarded me your article about your having had prostate surgery. I just read it. Gave me quite a chuckle. I too had THE surgery last December. I had no incontinence, but sexual recovery has yet to be fully experienced.

I like the grandeur in that sentence.

I have Viagra but have not tried it yet. My PSA is .49. My doctor says I may have to have radiation if it goes to .7 or .8. Like you, I'm glad I had the surgery . . . I just wanted to thank you for your humor. That's sometimes the biggest help through this kind of thing.

Humor is the best tonic, somebody said, and they would be right.

I received this from a fellow journalist on August 23, 2001:

like you, (I) had an RP at a young age (48 at the time, now 50). I applaud you for your honesty and forthrightness. My own experience is that we talk a lot about RP but not enough about the effects. My surgeon was spare in his comments. "You will be fine in six months," he said. He said nothing specific about leaking, erections, (or) the gap between the brain and groin (libido). One of the things that fascinates me intellectually (and yes is occasionally depressing) is that when I see a pretty woman, the physical response simply doesn't kick in. This is all about nerves and chemicals.

Or lack of them—see Chapter 9.

But they don't talk so much about that . . . I know some folks thought it was a provocative piece. I thought it was great.

In late 2008 he wrote again with the news that he was fine, and on track in all respects.

Another Steve emerged from the *Post* readership to offer this:

You wrote a true and very descriptive article which all prospective patients should be required to read!

Once, again, I would reply to Steve that it's pretty sad that my article had the impact it did. I would have been much happier had there been so much awareness of the effects of prostate cancer and its treatments that my article had been summarily rejected by the *Post* and the other newspapers that expressed interest. Steve had this to say:

> *I had the surgery 3/5/01 and have experienced almost identical residual effects as you. I still have some problems inflating but at 58 possibly age may be an issue. I have noticed that with Viagra I do not inflate quite as hard but as my wife has major vaginal discomfort during sex the old hand, Rosie Palm, does a reasonable job.*

Too bad this Steve didn't write a book. I'd have read it, though I doubt his wife would have. "Vaginal discomfort?" I've never heard that one before. He added:

> *The best part is knowing that the cancer is gone! I will pass on copies of your article to my surgeon and anyone else who is contemplating this procedure.*

Al wrote to me August 23, 2001, nine days after the article first appeared:

> *Last year my PSA shot up over 3 points between two routine annual physicals and it took five months of additional testing and treatment before the possibility of cancer was eliminated. Even though I was 64 at the time, the idea of facing an altered or even an end to an active sex life was a major concern.*

Atta boy, Al!

> *I know men that have had surgery, as you have had, but did not feel comfortable in asking them how their equipment was working for them. Brave souls like you that are willing to share your experiences do more to help those of us facing this possibility than the words of the urologist and their nurses trying to reassure us. Yes, the bloody ejaculate experienced after the biopsy was nothing like the "little blood in the semen" the nurse warned me about. You shared what was real, not some vague possibility in this example as well as other experiences.*

There's enough vagueness in the world; the last thing I want to do is contribute to it.

Leave it to senior citizen Dick to inform us of the dangers of not getting follow-up treatment after surgery:

> *Just finished reading your report. I am 77 years old and went through the same thing about eight years ago . . . About a month ago my primary physician*

> *asked if I was seeing my urologist. I told him I hadn't. He said there is something that should be checked out . . . The surgeon reprimanded me for not checking in with him regularly. I replied that he told me the surgery would eliminate the cancer. He said I was mistaken. My reading had gone from 2.0 to 4.3. I was informed that after surgery that reading is too high. Once more I could disregard treatment, as one doctor suggested, or go through hormone shots (one every 3 months for 18 months) plus radiation, and daily pills. My brother (15 years younger), who also has the problem, advised me to go through with the whole enchilada. His surgery left him incontinent, and he is still under treatment . . . It took me a long time to learn that it was possible to have a sexual climax.*

Talk about bad communication!

> *The doctors must be too embarrassed to be frank about sex. I was given a video tape on a device that could be inflated over the penis. I thought it was ridiculous. I never considered Viagra. Sex is not that important at my age. I feel a closeness with my wife stronger than ever. My purpose in replying to you is to tell you to get regular check-ups.*

Fear still had a hold on Dick even after the surgery. I guess Dick was not familiar with the idea of "in for a penny, in for a pound."

I reprint the following e-mail to me with a warning. The writer, Neal Deoul, is the prime advocate of a controversial prostate cancer treatment using cesium. I have no opinion on this treatment, nor does the publisher.

> *I very much enjoyed reading your "colorful" August 14th article in the* Washington Post *detailing your experiences with prostate cancer. How unfortunate that you were never referred to my website www.cancer-coverup.com by your urologist prior to surgery. Of course he would have lost a surgical fee, but you, like me, would have been spared your ordeal. It's amazing how no one in the cancer industry wants people like you to know that cesium, nature's most alkaline element, is a very effective, natural (i.e. inexpensive) cancer killer, with virtually no side effects . . . I sincerely hope you have continued, total success with your decision because anyone who can express himself as well as you can deserves only the best!*

Even to this day, there is little information available about the treatment Deoul refers to, which is not the Cesium 131 seeds treatment. Admittedly, although I am open-minded about treatment options for others, I would not have looked into this "soft" approach when surgical alternatives were available to me.

Doug wrote to me on August 20, 2001:

> *I just discovered that I have an early stage (PSA 4.6 and Gleason 6) of prostate cancer and I am still trying to decide if I want to have surgery or seed implants. I am 63 years old and in good physical condition so I have the same concerns that you did. It is tough making such a decision when all you have to read are medical journals or books written by doctors who are biased one way or the other . . . My greatest fear is incontinence and it seems there is more risk in the surgery. I would greatly appreciate it if you could help me with this decision. Again, thank you for this candid article.*

A determined guy named Herman, whose erectile nerves were not spared, recommended pelvic floor muscle exercises for urine leakage. I'd never tried this, nor did Fred ever mention anything about it. I will say that when I try to do sit-ups, I am prone to leakage. For spontaneous sex, Herman uses MUSE (medicated urethral suppository for erection), "*inserted into the head of the penis. It works. Erection occurs in 10–15 minutes.*" Again, I have no experience with MUSE, and thus have no opinion about it. If you're curious, go to http://mens-health.health-cares.net/impotence-muse.php. Herman also uses erectile rings and KY gel. Where there's a will . . .

Another young cancer patient was Bob, who wrote to me on August 18, 2001:

> *I am also a young prostate cancer surgery patient (44, surgery November 1999) and I could fully relate to your article. I found your article to be painfully accurate. I have found it extremely difficult to share my experiences with my 40 year old peers because most of them are "clueless" about their prostate, ED or impotence. And most of the articles or books that have been written were by and for older men. So thanks for the article. I think there are many under 50 men who appreciated it . . . It's important for men to know that although they may still remain potent, they will have some form of ED. And there are a lot of emotions that will follow.*

Yes, something approaching a torrent.

Steven from New York had a story to tell that angered me, as he fell victim to charlatans in the treatment field:

> *I'm the same age as you and was diagnosed with Gleason 6 in June, 1999. I have been coaxed and harassed by my urologist ever since to have a radical. Unlike you, in the fall of 1999 I chose the herbal route with PC-SPES as the cornerstone and a host of other supplements.*

If for some reason you're interested in this largely debunked treatment, you can read about it here: http://altmedicine.about.com/cs/govtregulation/a/PCSpes.htm. I hope Steven saw the light in time, glinting off his urologist's scalpel.

Here's Julie, with some nice things to say:

your account of your experience with prostate cancer is so like my boyfriend's I just had to write to you. Like you he is young, 45, and our relationship is just passing the two year mark. . . . His cancer was discovered last October and his surgery was last December . . . He has become very open and vocal about his cancer, for which I thank you. For him and other men it is a difficult thing to do.

Years ago, yes, I might have had difficulty speaking and writing about such an ordeal, but several brushes with death have removed all reluctance.

Then there was a *Post* reader who didn't sign her rather lengthy note to me, yet it may be the best of the large batch I received. A brief excerpt:

My husband opted for seed implants and radiation, rejecting an earlier decision to have a radical prostatectomy. This choice was driven by concerns of possible escaped cancer cells due to the location of the cancer . . . Some of your thoughts echo what I have heard my husband say about his sexual changes and urinary urgency and frequency . . . His comment has been "I'm sure glad I'm not dating, how would I explain this?" . . . What is gone from his attitude is his assured cockiness that you describe in your article . . . Because it is not my body that has been assaulted and insulted it has been easier for me than him to accept different standards of sexual functioning than before his treatments. From the female perspective, I assure you no gratitude is needed or wanted for accepting the changes in sexual performance.

A woman in love is the most amazing creature on earth.

If this were a modern romance novel the heroine would contrive an experiment by managing to allow her mate to explore sexually with others, to learn just how desirable he is, how little women care about the different responses you describe after surgery. . . . My husband will have to get over his changed perceptions without the intervention of any stray vixens.

Love this woman, whoever she is! She went on to say that one night, after using Viagra, her husband passed out in the bathroom and hit his head, requiring stitches. Readers: Any strong drug that alters your blood flow should be taken with care. Whenever you stand from a reclining position, be aware of Viagra's potential to cause dizziness and loss of consciousness.

Then there's this anonymous guy. I like his style:

I liked that article you wrote . . . I just went through that same operation on the 28th of November 2000. My operation didn't go as well but all is well now. I am 64 and back to playing golf. Thank God for Viagra, it works.

You get the impression he put down his putter just long enough to tap out those words. Good for him. I wish I could play golf without being obsessed about it. I shot an 86 once, but I know what it would take to become good . . . too much time. Maybe when I'm in my 60s, with my buddy Tom, who plays three times week these days, when there's no snow on the ground in Connecticut . . .

Returning to the ranks of those who enjoy traditional social intercourse, which all cultures deem superior to being merely in touch with oneself, sometimes I'm not so sure one and one is better than one, as solitude in this technological age can be liberating. I pity young men who have to keep the attention of young girls these days. The distractions are 10 times what they were when I was in my 20s. TV is the least of it. The glamour anxiety induced by women's magazines is a pernicious element that wreaks havoc with relationships just when a young person's identity is most fragile.

The fashion and cosmetics industries conspire with big media to drive young women to extremes of insecurity. Vapidity becomes an asset in the role models of Paris Hilton, Lindsey Lohan and Britney Spears who, on camera, seem bent on destroying their self-respect. The trend is toward sleaze, and although this tendency does not bother me per se, with rare exception there is no mature eroticism on TV today. There was a wildly erotic scene in HBO's *Rome*, but that's pay-TV, the last refuge for adults with a liberal attitude toward sex. Of course this may be because we are, comparatively, a nation of unread, self-absorbed blockheads, but then again, maybe not. But for the most part we take our natural resources and our economic power, for granted. And yet the unfortunate man with prostate cancer in America may be so discouraged that he doesn't even bother to get a diagnosis. Only when he is broken apart by metastases does he make it to the hospital for endgame palliative treatment.

I fear for the collective mental health of the generation now in their teens and 20s. Make no mistake, it's all about sex. Girls think to themselves "Am I good enough? Does he want me? If not, why not?" This is the culture that I staggered back into after surgery. Women of all ages think "What can I do to get him to want me?" Forget about the spiritual components of self-improvement that lead to attracting the opposite sex—not that looks will ever play a diminished role. In modern America, the talentless skank rules our attention-whore mindset, as young people jockey to catch a glimpse of the next "hot mess," that B- or C-list celeb hellbent on becoming the next Anna Nicole Smith. Shame needs to make a comeback in America, and soon. One cannot have dignity without the potential for shame, as they are two sides of the same coin.

Back in early 2000, it meant a great deal to me to be able to make love again, to be made whole, as it were, although emotionally I lagged months behind my body's renewed readiness for naked undulations. Thankfully, I wasn't dragging much personal or cultural baggage along with me, as I've worked carefully over the years to shed the ubiquitous influences borne on the dark wings of the media, with which I have a love/hate relationship. At least as much as the next guy, I enjoy a Victoria's Secret TV special, but to be bombarded for years on end with images of sexually attractive females who are out of reach must have taken a significant toll on my subconscious.

What about men who are unaware of the grinding toll taken on them? How many men act out immorally, if not criminally, because of this relentless media barrage? It's probably easier on the straight male psyche to stroll the streets of Teheran, as opposed to Miami Beach, women's rights notwithstanding. Recall those years in the 1980s, when all the psychologists were touting the idea of rape as a pure power crime? True, some men rape because they wish to exert power over the women they hate. But just as often, in my opinion, men rape because they can't get sex another way. It can be as simple as that. Academic studies often fail to measure common sense.

Back in New York, I had sponsored another A.A. member who was arrested for sexual assault. He spent six months in jail before I saw him again. I asked him why he attacked the girl. He said, "She wouldn't give it up," with an expression that indicated he was disappointed at the extent of my stupidity. My point here is that there is a whole layer of male reality that goes unmeasured and unaddressed, except in prison, where behavior is interpreted to meet the clinical norms of the moment.

Imagine the deconstruction of our dating culture to the point where a guy sits his date down for dinner and commences with "Hi. I asked you out tonight because I want to have sex with you. I don't want to talk to you, but I understand I may have to listen for a while to appear as if I'm interested in what you have to say. We have nothing in common and so the only reason for us to meet is to have sex. If you delay this process or act in a passive-aggressive manner, I am likely to take out my aggressions on you or someone like you. What would you like to drink?"

This is what goes on in the minds of countless men when they're out on a date. So few women, despite the myriad crime shows on TV, understand the depth and strength of the male id. Many women who have survived assaults by mismanaged male ids say they wish they hadn't survived. I see such women in the rooms of A.A. all the time. And don't even get me started on the incidence of incest in this country. Its prevalence is as disgusting as the behavior itself.

As for those men who enjoy strip clubs, you have only my sympathy. I would no sooner watch a pole dance than I would gaze upon a scrumptious buffet without chowing down. Alas, the creature that passes for the normal American male often cultivates a masochistic streak in himself, so the phenomena of this kind of craving should not be too discouraging. I recall the words of a New Orleans hooker during Mardi Gras in 1978, referring to men, "There's hope for you bastards yet." I bought her another scotch, but given her mangy looks, more than my moral standards, I bought nothing more.

So in 2000, it was my personal baggage, not the insecurities generated by media images or miscues in my past, that underpinned my feelings. More recently, however, reflections on the activity of penises connected to men younger and more fortunate than myself have incurred brief periods of wonderment, if not prolonged contemplation. And the media is again, in my opinion, to blame. New England Patriots' Quarterback Tom Brady comes to mind. Where he has been, all straight men yearn to follow. Sure, I may have enjoyed my share of beautiful women over the years, but guys like Brady are upsetting nature's balance. Tom Brady must be stopped! Watching him beat the Eagles, the other day, I thought to myself: The definition of Tom Brady getting annoyed is, he has to get up somewhat early on a Sunday morning, abandoning the wifey, Giselle Bundchen, naked under the comforter, so he can meet his obligations on the football field. Maybe she whips up some scrambled eggs for him first.

Still, in 2000 I looked forward to decades of satisfying sack time. But getting my sexual confidence back has not been straightforward as, for the first two years of my recovery, when anxiety, a most familiar demon, crept into my mind, my penis would abandon all skyward pretense. I comfort myself with the thought that Tom Brady will get old someday, too. In the meantime I applaud his ability to appear as if his liaisons with the likes of Bridget Moynihan and Ms. Bundchen matter not a bit to him. What's that joke about the old bull and the young bull standing on a hilltop overlooking a valley full of cows? The old bull says something about "Forget running—let's walk down there and mount 'em all." Most of us are happy to find the right woman.

It's reasonable to predict that most readers of this book will be in their 50s and 60s, an age when most men will have settled into a less edgy sexuality compared to that of younger men. I, for one, am relieved to be less driven to copulate. Enough of the constant pressure already! Three decades was enough. Yet one must be careful not to get too comfortable about that, for there are few sources of reassurance that won't take your money with a rueful smile. Once the testosterone level diminishes, so much mental energy is freed up to concentrate on other things; plus, the role of indentured servant to one's libido is most gratefully terminated. Of course, some days I yearn for that feral feeling of 20 years ago, when I often felt little separated from the beasts of the forest.

Recalling those days, it is laughable that I was a proud owner of what I thought was free will. In reality, my choices were severely narrowed by hormonal variables. These forces were more subtle than the power of my conscious mind to focus on any given subject. Philosophically, this is comforting, for I can readily count myself as among the vast majority of people who live in delusion, in one altered state or another, while thinking they are high-order mammals of pure choice. As I age, I learn that freedom is not so simple a concept, and I deeply resent those who taught me it was a simple idea when I was very young, especially while trying to inculcate me with fear-mongering Christianity.

So it comes as no surprise to the reader that we are all slaves to innumerable impulses and drives, even if we do not act on them, so much so that I find it hard to imagine what pure freedom might be like. Perhaps a blind eunuch would have some idea, as the first step in that discovery would be to be neutered, but as I stand back, legs together, and consider the ramifications, I'm not that curious. Besides, I don't have the looks for a fresh career as a soprano. Better I continue to suffer the consequences of my knuckle-dragging ways and get on with it.

One benefit of a less aggressive sex drive is that one may be aware of women's true spiritual preferences without filtering, coalescing in the mind without the id playing havoc with thought processes. And what of men's preferences? Most every straight man has been struck stupid by some female who may not even be likeable, yet her vise-grip on him, enforced by the hairy hand of millions of years of evolution, can be both unrelenting and merciless. At times, the only two options may appear to be: surrender to the magnetism and marry the girl or flee the country. However, there is no safe quarter from, or statute of limitations on, such feelings. And both options may, from time to time, seem equally appealing, depending on how the woman in question treats you.

Women may have chuckled at 89-year-old billionaire Howard Marshall's marriage to Anna Nicole Smith, but men stayed silent. We know that what works on us when we're 18 works when we're 89, unless a specific woman has endeared herself to us through the tools of charm at her disposal. When I was 18, did I care about a girl's ability to cook? No, of course not. Not until recently did such domestic capabilities factor in at all in my personal equation. When I was 18, a girl's name was superfluous, and I don't consider myself unusual in that respect, although in the lily-white town in which I grew up, one had to be very careful to accord girls the equal status they deserved. But I recall wanting them, and little more. Not a single shred of conversation with a girl from my teen years survives in my memory, although I remember the physical characteristics of many of them quite precisely, down to the quivering bridge of saliva that linked a certain brunette's perfect white teeth.

Back in Hollywood in the early spring of 2000, months had passed without an erection, for me, anyway. I'm sure they were springing up all over my Hollywood neighborhood, which is full of hottie actresses and wide-eyed Scientologist magazine models eager to dispense the favors attendant on their nonexistent self-esteem. I felt somewhat like the lonely soldier who sits in a hut in northern Canada, riveted on a radar screen for weeks on end, hoping against hope for a Russian nuke to appear as a blip, shaking up his existence forever. Oh, for a bulge in my pants!

In those early recovery days, there seemed to be no point in mere socializing, as urinary continence was still sketchy. I learned to avoid tea, which seemed to run right through me. I prefer decaf coffee anyway. Still, at the time, I was bowling in a couple leagues per week, so I did what I had to do to make the commitments to my teams, especially in the scratch league, where scoring was taken seriously. Running to the men's room every few hours became routine. In 2000, I would have had to go maybe six times per day.

My surgical scar had gradually turned from angry purple to red and then to pink. I should have taken that improvement as an indicator of the healing going on inside me as well, but I was too distraught from misplaced musings about my future to make the connection. Emotionally, the choices were to capitulate to depressive feelings or keep my faith in Fred Kuyt, who had promised me that firmness would return in time. Patience. Indeed, this can be true for many, if not for most of us overloaded with technology. Most of the time I like the fast pace of modern life, but when my penis was overcooked, shall I say, life looked quite gray most of the time. I could laugh at myself, but not for long. Friends, Debbie, and A.A. meetings helped me reset my goal-oriented bearings.

Just because I was temporarily infirm in one area didn't mean everything else had to shut down. I knew that, but getting myself motivated was difficult. There had been times in years past when the clinical depression was so strong I would sit up in bed with plans for the day, yet all I could do was feel tears run down my cheeks. I was paralyzed and overwhelmed. The sense of dread from swimming in thoughts of "what's the point?" was so bleak and pervasive I cannot frankly recall the depth of those torments today. My introduction to Lexapro would come in 2004, years down the road.

Thus, relaxation, from where I sat then or sit today, is an art form not yet in my skill set. I haven't been on a true vacation in 20 years because there's not much point to it. During those first six months of recovery, if I hadn't had books and bowling in which to lose myself, I'd have gone more than a bit crazy. I've tried meditation, but I always feel I am missing the possibly of an original idea if I clear my head of thoughts. Orgasm is the only mental obliteration I welcome today, now that booze and drugs are off limits. So sex is important to me on that level too, as a refuge from the demands of pedestrian life and logic. Sure, sex has its own logic, but it never feels like its mine; it feels rather borrowed from a hidden source to be provisionally trusted, God perhaps. Moreover, sex gives us the Pavlovian assurance that it will always work, despite the fact that, next to greed, it screws up more lives than any other behavior in the human spectrum. I had contented myself for what seemed like 100-day months with what the Bible calls onanism, although that popular book mentions nothing about erectile dysfunction. On second thought, maybe it does. I haven't read it in awhile.

In the last 20 years or longer, I've read that mood and attitude play a big part in cancer recovery. This made sense to me, as someone whose often grim take on life had caused ulcers, skin rashes and other maladies. Lately, though, there seems to be evidence to the contrary, as a 2007 study of 1,000-plus subjects indicated that mood has no effect on the progress of cancer or its treatment. So should one feel free to rant and rave at the moon for the injustice of it all? The study results support the proposition that cancer sufferers' lives are not lengthened by group sharing or other less structured forms of hand-holding, including holding one's own hand in counsel with a higher power. I would like to think that applied science, not group hugs, offers whatever hope we have for treatment and recovery. Still, hugs are critical, at any time, for anyone. Shared emotions are one of life's great joys. Was it me who just typed that sentence? Remarkable.

If cancer is ever cured, it will likely be as a result of the zillions of dollars and zillions of academic research hours put into the effort, not because some guru laid on hands. My point here is that prayers go unheard as well. If that idea offends you, I would pray for you if I thought it would work. I especially address these harsh, anti-religious sentiments to those of you who have prostate cancer but are waiting to see what happens because you think God is on your side. You may think that God will intervene and spare you a painful death. The popular TV pastor Dr. Gene Scott, with all of his Biblical erudition, apparently felt his striving to know the nature of God through Jesus was enough to stave off the ravages of prostate cancer. God, if there is one out there, took no notice, and Dr. Scott succumbed just as we all would if we don't take full responsibility for our condition. Someday far in the future, the majority of mankind will take full responsibility for their own lives.

The report cited previously, published in the October 2007 issue of the journal *Cancer*, found that patients with a cheerful attitude had the same life expectancy as those who were miserable. This report cheers me up, as yet another example of reflecting man's arrogance in thinking that will alone can determine outcomes. Didn't Hitler teach us anything about unchecked will and where it leads? Now, I'm not arguing against keeping one's chin up through adversity, but in the annals of behavioral etiquette, the stiff upper lip was implemented for the benefit of others, not the sufferer himself. One cancer researcher, Dr. Janice Kiecolt-Glaser, has said regarding the link between cancer and emotions: "If a freight train is coming it doesn't matter how many people stand in front of it, nothing is going to stop it." That analogy is a few degrees off, but you get her point. Similarly, James Coyne, lead author of the recent cancer/emotion longevity study, said "if you attend a support group in the belief that you are increasing your chances of survival, you are going to be disappointed." He gets points for understatement.

So given that this study has granted the cancer-afflicted man permission for an occasional bout of misery, as an adult in his 50s, I find myself effortlessly attracted to women who are certainly feminine and intelligent, but also tough minded. The TV character that comes to mind as a paradigm of this type of woman is Diane Russell, the cop played by Kim Delaney on *NYPD Blue*. Her sexiness is a byproduct of going about her business as a goal-oriented professional. A nice face and good body help, but unless a woman has an air of competence, I can't get too interested. I also love the Lisa Cuddy character played by Lisa Edelstein on *House, M.D.* It doesn't much matter to me what a woman is competent at, but she's got to be good at something that interweaves her personality into the fabric of either the artistic community or business or social services. It is the rare young woman who understands this, and by merely preening for hours in front of the mirror only to stand in line to get into a club, all many women are doing is labeling themselves as insubstantial.

As I age, my conscious mind becomes more in control of what I want, and when and how I act, in all areas. And yet sometimes the id rises out of the gloom to make itself known as the powerful force that it is. Reconsidering the id makes me uncomfortable, for I have gone to great lengths over the years to tame it. How to characterize this dark force that makes us do crazy things? This is the force that makes people obsess, stalk, kill, and otherwise engage in all sorts of horrible thought processes and behaviors. Have you ever been hopelessly in lust after a woman with whom you have nothing in common, to the point where you cannot sleep or work effectively? Despite the fact that she may be selfish and mean, you feel you would cut off a finger to spend a weekend in bed with her. The id runs through all of us as a common thread that draws its power from some mechanism that makes us akin to reptiles and other driven creatures. Whole religions have been formed as systems of denial of the id, yet as many wayward priests have proven, the id often expresses itself despite the best intentions to curtail it.

Thus, anything that man spends so much time fighting is of endless fascination to me, even if I am personally in its grip. Conversely, who has not had a friend who marries a woman no other man within 50 miles finds the least bit attractive? Such attraction has nothing to do with conscious choice. We are overcome with feelings so inexplicable that there is hell to pay if they are not managed effectively. If we are fortunate, the object of such desire is a nice person and wants us in return. In lieu of that, we should welcome her rejection if she is a nice person, as the depth of wanting may be beyond healthy norms. Worst case, she returns our panting entreaties and is a mean and vengeful type with a history of abuse. In such cases we'd be better off taking up bull-riding as a pastime. Much safer.

I have at times been so overcome by this id-driven craving that I will write a book dedicated to it, in the form of a 300-page letter to a particular woman, explaining my irrational feelings. Thankfully, I have developed a productive outlet for expressing my id, and in writing the "letter" I hope to learn a great deal about my innermost self. I can't say I'm looking forward to writing it, but it's something I must do to gain self-knowledge. If there were another way to explore and get through the feelings (which seems like such an inadequate catch-all word) in a cleansing way, I would do it. I have tried talking to her, but her insouciance informs me she's heard it all before, which of course only makes me feel worse. Doesn't she comprehend that my feelings are unique and not to be trifled with, frustrating to the point where I threaten to end sentences with a preposition? I'll cut myself off here about this issue, lest I start writing the next book here. It's too easy to get riled up about it. Damn id. Thankfully, Debbie understands that my mind goes off on these tangents from time to time. My mind's travel plans are no reflection on her, that's for sure. She has been wonderful to me, and for me.

Six months along into my post-op recovery, I was able to have sex somewhat normally, after displaying a few dozen test erections for no one's entertainment but my own. Yet finally the time came to share. With the help of Viagra, my penis achieved a one-towel rating around this time, in the spring of 2000, sufficiently firm to reclaim its rightful place in the realm of delight. I didn't put it quite that way to Debbie, although she has endured my waxing grandiloquent plenty of times.

Timing being half of luck in life, she was not around when my penis was initially resurrected from the scrap heap of dead members of the flesh. I recall one morning when, reminiscent of morning erections of the adolescent variety, I welcomed my tumescent friend. Mr. Harry Swelling was back, unpacking his bag! Welcome home! With a sigh of relief, I rolled over and slept again, perhaps more deeply than in months. Around noon, I woke up again to reaffirm my grip and to bring it to one-towel status, thanks to visuals provided by several nameless babes in Telemundo's telenovellas. I love those pouty-lipped Latin girls on those sickly sweet melodramas, and wonder where they hide during the day.

Toward orgasm that afternoon, I was presented with a serviceable erection, which triggered a phone call to Debbie with the good news.

"That's great," she said, as if she knew it was an eventuality.

Buoyed, I went grocery shopping with a new bounce in my step and a melody in my heart. My depression lifted a great deal.

Maybe I'm being too harsh on those who have found their own way in dealing with "fear and trembling unto death," as the King of Bleak, philosopher Søren Kierkegaard, put it. I was raised a Protestant, but that belief system was easy to dismiss as a contraption dependent on man's imagination and the yearning for immortality. Cancer brings these feelings to a head, even if one's prognosis is good. Certainly, six months after my operation, I was in no way convinced that I was cured. I spent hours of quiet time conjuring the most diabolical end that a God might devise, before realizing that perfect indifference ruled the day, as usual, even if God did exist. My investment was in man and his tenuous grasp on science and the natural world. I would keep my bond with the medical community, despite my political leanings toward universal health coverage.

It's easy for me to imagine men out there reading this book in libraries, knowing they have prostate cancer, yet not having the means to pay for surgery or other treatment. If so, I have a suggestion. Go to your local newspaper and find a liberal reporter who is willing to follow you around as you approach hospitals in an effort to get the surgery. To be effective, leverage your personality so that hospital administrators see the benefits in performing the procedure on you. This may sound farfetched, but make no mistake, if I had to, I'd have gotten very creative. Maybe you'll end up owing the hospital for their services. Get it done any way you can. Think about showing up at the emergency room claiming you're going to die if you don't get surgery. It is true, even if your death is years off. Hospital personnel will have to scramble to find a way to get rid of you without leaving themselves open to legal action. I'm not advocating anarchy, but shyness in the face of potentially terminal illness makes no sense at all. Another idea would be to offer yourself up as a subject at a teaching hospital. Maybe a college-aligned facility would perform the surgery if you permit a throng of gawking medical students to watch. Or move to Canada, a more civilized nation with universal healthcare. Get creative if you cannot afford treatment, and don't assume everyone you approach will say no. There is power in boldness alone, to paraphrase Goethe. If you don't ask, you don't get, to quote my friend, the less well-known philosopher Mike Vietro.

Returning to Debbie's arms was reassuring, as my erectile ability was tenuous. No surprise there. My mind was embattled. Memories of multi-towel pre-op erections were fresh, yet I had to be grateful for the one-toweler that was gaining me reentry to the pleasure dome.

Those initial forays went well. Debbie and I resumed the familiar rhythms that have both promulgated the species and kept the genders close. Yet it wasn't the sex itself that lifted me up, but rather the sense of having healed. With my dark emotional background, I am susceptible to feelings that induce a sense of redemption, including the physical sort. I am so sensitive to this trait in others that I can spot people who do not have it. Those are the ones who smile and look like they know they will not only live forever, but live forever vitally. What a gift that is. But be extra grateful if that describes you. You know the bell will one day toll for you, and if you have prostate cancer, mortality is most likely in the front of your mind. Even so, I know better than to exhort those who are simply afraid of going forward with treatment. What's to become of you?

Eight

USERS' MANUAL

Perhaps it's ironic to thank ex-New York governor Eliot Spitzer for providing such a superb example of a man expressing his innermost nature. Consider what was on each side of his decision seesaw before he blew up his career. On one side was his stellar career, forged on the do-gooder anvil. He has or had a lovely wife and two teenaged daughters who seemingly loved and admired him. He had money, power and the kind of fame that is more manageable than the Hollywood sort. Ostensibly, he had a nearly perfect, fulfilling life. On the other side, in the form of a hooker with the working name Kristen, stood, or rather reclined, apex fecundity. She was at her peak as a uterine magnet for male energy. Even with all the intellectual and psychological resources at his command, Spitzer chose apex fecundity over a rich, stable life, solidly proving the point that the outcome of five million years of evolutionary wiring can still be choices most feral, even when there is everything to lose. Kristen, not the most fragile or girly of specimens, has a sturdy femininity about her that speaks of the irresistible force that would have Darth Vader cowering, fully reflected in the $4,300 fee attached to her facilities. Spitzer may have been an idiot to consort with her, but an idiot who nonetheless got what he truly wanted. What price satisfaction? Meanwhile, illegal prostitution thrives as a multi-billion dollar industry in the United States, making criminals of women who are disallowed from leveraging their primary assets in activities between consenting adults.

The story of the ex-governor has broad [sic.] implications to men recovering from prostate cancer surgery. Trust me. For guys who are unattached, the menu of female choices may change due to diminished erectile capacity. And there is the likelihood that one's personality will change to reflect alterations in sexual plumbing. As anxiety takes hold, the bold extrovert may become a reticent introvert. The lucky ones will emerge with their integrated personalities intact, assuming that sociability is part of their makeup before surgery. Most men will be affected to a lesser degree. The most fortunate won't lose a step, as their identities will not have been tied to erectile ability. I say to such guys: I don't know whether to admire or pity you.

Still, if you are out in the dating world, look to—perhaps—get reacquainted with anxiety levels you were fully convinced vacated your mind after high school. As a survivor, there is a sequence of disclosures you will face as potential relationships grow. Every guy will have to find their particular comfort zone in revealing to his dates when to spring the news that: (1) I cannot perform the way I once could; (2) I no longer emit semen; (3) it still feels pretty much the same when stimulated, and (4) don't worry, you're not going to break anything. Or, you could omit Step 1, since most women are unlikely to be interested in things you *used to* be able to do. Women are often that way, practical thinkers as most of them are. If you were a high school football hero whose six-pack has long since migrated from your abs to your tailgate cooler, she will likely ask you to save your stories of gridiron heroics for your buddies.

In my mind, as I was writing this book over several years in my spare time, I keep returning to the robust erections I had achieved prior to surgery, not a big deal for anyone but me, but then again, this was a personal barometer of good health on which I had banked most of my wavering self-confidence. For me, once a few years had elapsed since my surgery, the challenge became to settle into a routine of making consistently positive decisions, somewhat as a substitute for my former erection-based confidence. I had to rebuild my sense of self on a more spiritual foundation and, frankly, I wasn't too happy about it. This is probably because I am especially resistant to being forced by circumstances to alter my behavior. I hate most holidays, for example. And it's very tough to tell a clinically depressed person that any of his freedoms are being changed against his will. Since about 2005, however, my sex drive has waned (see next chapter), so since then such rebuilding has no longer carried with it any resentment about my firmer past.

Patience takes on a twisted quality when it's forced upon you by infirmity. One's mind races ahead of one's body and there is that privately humiliating period when your body tries to catch up. Sometimes it gets there, sometimes not. One is encouraged to accept age-related changes that cannot be reversed, or craziness can quickly set in. The mind may play tricks on you that cannot be anticipated, so be kind to yourself and roll with it, as they say. I hope many of you don't know what I'm writing about here, as you are the type to adjust naturally to change. Good for you. But there are, conversely, many guys who will never adjust to the changes I'm writing about. You are the ones I want most to reach. For you, it's good to apply a maxim I learned 25 years ago: Good feelings follow good actions. It's like getting over the mental block to exercise. You know it's good for you, yet getting out there and doing it may require breaking through the bondage of self. That can be the most difficult task we face.

I came to accept the phenomenon of slow-motion erections, relative to my presurgery days. There was planning involved, not on the scale of rebuilding at Ground Zero, perhaps, but along the lines of planning a picnic. Everything had to be packed and laid out to be enjoyed by those involved. Yet when the Viagra kicked in, erections were firm and serviceable. Sometimes, when well-rested and in a calm frame of mind, I can achieve erections that enable penetration without Viagra. Men who enjoy a more peaceful mindset will certainly enjoy a more favorable result than I do, and perhaps not need Viagra or Cialis or other erectile drugs at all. If that's your experience, great. I'm mildly jealous. I have always had a fevered mind, and it often works to my detriment, though it was helpful when my sex drive waned, as lower testosterone levels bode well for male sanity.

Ah, lost youth! How miserable I was in my 20s. I just didn't give a damn. My hormone- and drug-addled friends and I used to joke about a common movie theme, the one about girls complaining about being used for sex. Some of our attitude was a hangover from being subjected to *Love Story,* which was saccharine schlock of the first order. That film's key line, "Love means never having to say you're sorry," didn't make any sense then, and it makes less sense now. In our minds, the line may have evolved into something like "Love means never having to say 'I love you'," or, in certain situations, "Love means not being able to say anything—because you're gagged with a red rubber ball." That's a love story I could relate to then, but not today. Young men try different things to establish their dominance in relationships and they keep trying until they find out what works. Women, meanwhile, know what tools they have and do their best to sharpen them. Chaos ensues. As TV's Dr. Drew Pinsky has said so wisely, "People in their twenties treat each other terribly."

By the time men are in their 20s, they've either figured out how to score, or they've turned to other pursuits, some healthy, some not. From our collective perspective in our 20s, girls were, in theory, multi-orgasmic, so in a typical romp, a woman might out-spasm her male partner five or even ten times to one in that life-affirming department. How can she say she's being used, when she's having the better time of it? we wondered. Men tend to keep score, but still, could we believe our girlfriends when they explained that what the films were hinting at had to do with a women's inherent sense of vulnerability in sexual situations? Therefore, once a guy had been permitted to traverse the great divide, his partner is open to being hurt if she isn't thoroughly reassured that she is either loved or at least respected in the morning. My response to this was practical. What a racket these girls have going! Not only are they wired for unlimited orgasms, they get to play the "hurt" card whenever they want. Back then, if a guy claimed to his friends that a girl had hurt his feelings, he might as well wear a skirt. The unspoken admonition in these circumstances was to find another girl to play with, since we understood that it's very tough to maintain hurt feelings about Maria while climaxing in the arms of Gina. (As you might have guessed, there were a lot of Italian girls in my hometown.)

This is an example of how cultural mores are established. Deflect human beings' natural drives and, in order to maintain law and order and establish Judeo-Christian repression, create an elaborate system of rules and etiquette that all good boys are forced to play by, or else. Consider the afternoon when two friends and I were aimlessly driving around town drinking beer. We were about 22 at the time. Back then MADD stood for Men Are Driving Drunk. I was in the back seat. We picked up a hitchhiker, a girl of 18 or 19, rough around the edges but cute. She looked like Squeaky Fromme, one of murder cult leader Charlie Manson's most devout followers. She wanted a ride to the north side of the next town, Danbury, perhaps 30 miles away. This was out of our way, which presumed of course, that we had somewhere important to go. I suggested she give us gas and beer money. She wasn't having it, so I suggested a more personal, manual favor. Again, if you don't ask, you don't get.

Guys like the barter system. In the fullness of the New England day, I proposed a release of sexual tension in exchange for a ride across Fairfield County. The girl had gotten into the car with an air of experience about her, so I figured if she took offense it would be expressed with the practiced histrionics she had learned from her mother. Understand that we were guys who hung around girls who measured the quality of their dates in a way that is too crude to describe in this book, so we would pretty much say anything and do almost anything. The word "no" held no pain in it, as that word fully embraced our low expectations. This is how we learn to hear "yes" as a pleasant surprise.

To the girl's credit, she activated the actuarial part of her brain and took a few seconds to think about the cost/reward equation. The hesitation told me she was from out of town, because if she were from our Republican burg, she'd have demanded immediate egress from the vehicle, lest the shame of even a brief consideration of such a wanton deed sully her day.

"All of you?" She hoped not.

"No, just me," I said, pressing the bet. It was presumed my buddies would watch or turn away, as they wished.

"Give me a beer," she said. We laughed and cracked her a cold one, which she drank in two or three gulps. Back then, prior to pop-tops, one kept a can opener or "church key" in the glove compartment.

"Come on," I pleaded. "You want us to drive you way the hell in the other direction, and I'm the one with no girlfriend." I was right back in the green rowboat of some years ago.

"Thanks for the beer, but no way. I don't do that kind of thing."

"You've never given a guy a hand-job before?"

"Well, yeah, but just my boyfriend."

"So pretend I'm your boyfriend until we get to Bethel," I said. I like rustic towns with a Biblical ring to them.

"No! Either you bastards give me a ride or let me out. I'll scream."

Great. I'm sure she made it to Bethel eventually, back when hitchhiking was relatively safe, even for girls. Arguments could be made to reflect changes in the negotiations. What if the hitchhiker wanted a 300-mile ride? What if I had leukemia and a handy was my dying wish? I knew a girl who claimed she had leukemia to get a lawyer's romantic attention. He laughed it off and told everyone in town. Of course, looking back, I'm not proud of this desperate mischief, but I cop to it anyway, for truth's sake. That was the worst of my sexual behavior.

What's the point of the hitchhiker story? Well, in each of life's phases our needs and priorities change, and this includes sex. Yet we don't hand prospective partners a users' manual, which would save everyone involved a lot of time and trouble, in my controversial opinion. In my youth, there were girls who understood that a hand job was a most effective intermediate step in inter-gender communications, and it was most often administered in a car. It was intimate, yet not really, as the friction was reserved for nonmucous membranes. For a hand-job, I would move furniture for a girl I didn't like or perform some other blue collar or car-related errand, again often for girls who did nothing for me in the romance department. I chased after the unattainable girls who were gorgeous and older than me, because I feared rejection from the girls my age. I could have typed up all my issues in a manual and handed it to a date, which, come to think of it, I never went out on, if you'll pardon the atrocious grammar. Dates were for normal guys who interpreted our evolutionary shift to bipedal status as progress.

Sex and Violence

Some readers will experience a shiver of anticipation as they commence reading this section. I hope they know why their hackles are raised. I include this brief look at the issue because the topic has been a major cause of distress for me over the years. Also, it is safe to assume that the subject has been a bane for many readers and the women they love. I am concerned about the brutality that goes on routinely behind closed doors in America, yet I am woefully uncertain what more can be done about it that is not being done presently. Western culture is full of people, men especially, who profess to hate abuse and violence. Yet the reality is that, for many men, violence is their primary mode of expression, and women are often their targets.

Does violence begin in the dark hearts of men or in our violence- and sex-obsessed culture? I was in London in the spring of 1972, when the X-rated Stanley Kubrick film *A Clockwork Orange* was in theatres. It was pandemonium in the streets for the repressed Brits, as they stood in long lines to get a taste of "the old ultra-violence," as the main character refers to it. The futuristic film was so ahead of its time it was banned in South Africa and in Ireland until 2000. Watch it today and it still has an impact, although current content on TV is more extreme.

Violence has become sexier than sex. How did that happen? I'm not talking about guys punching each other in the nose. Fistfights are as passé in film as they are in real life. A film antagonist must be eviscerated in order to get jaded film-goers' attention. Sitting in a movie theater, I often see unflinching 10-year-olds gobbling popcorn as characters are blown to bits or decapitated. Strength of story has taken a backseat to knife, gun and bomb-wielding savages driving the plotline forward—and I refer to the heroes. I suppose a psychologist would say that we need to see violence onscreen in order to achieve cathartic, psychic release at seeing characters do things to each other that real people cannot do with impunity.

I pause here in an either/or mindset about violence and sex in Western culture, as I tend to view them as polarized, not fused. How far can we, and our children, allow ourselves to be pushed in the direction of themes wherein sex and violence are indistinguishable? For the worst who walk among us in real life, they are the same. Not that I'm any sort of saint, but I know I've never hit a woman, which stems largely from what I saw inflicted on my mother by my father, although my mother had a big part in their ugly dynamic. My moral code draws a firm line at laying a hand on women, no matter how angry I get.

Thus, I have expended a lot of energy over three-quarters of a lifetime trying to do the opposite of what my old man did. Down very deep, I realize I chose not to have children for fear of repeating his mistakes. Of course, these old scars are at the core of my story. Violence is powerful stuff and I have no appetite for it at all in real life. In films and on TV, I can take it or leave it. When I hear male acquaintances admit to having abused their wives or girlfriends, I greet their expressed remorse with doubt, and view them in shadow ever after.

Is depicting sex in film so disturbing to Americans that violence is preferable? The culture says yes. In London, after *A Clockwork Orange* premiered, hoodlums took to the streets imitating the exploits of antihero Alex DeLarge, the key character who is both protagonist and antagonist, depending on one's take. One of the film's many themes is how desensitized we have become to violence in media. At the time, most adults found the film shocking. Today, the film's content would hardly merit cultural comment, underscoring the film's point. There is no theoretical limit to how far art can go with this subject and, for me, the line has already been crossed in the film *Happiness*. There's a profoundly disturbing scene in the last act where the pedophilic father in the story admits to his pre-pubescent son that he fantasizes about him sexually, and that he would act on it if given a chance. Despite having studied the depths of human depravity, from Hitler to de Sade to every more modern malefactor you could name, that scene rips me apart.

In order to generate discussion about sexual violence against women, I have devised the following quiz to shed light on the contrast between male and female perspectives.

Quiz

Women readers, do you think you know the nature of the human male animal? Here are some hypothetical scenarios for you to ponder. Critics quick to condemn may point out that I am not a licensed psychologist or psychiatrist. I respond by admitting to the fact that I am just a well-read layman. Even so, I ask readers to consider the following and draw your own conclusions:

1) A half-hour after sunset, deep in hunting country, a 20-something heterosexual male sits in a small town coffee shop, reading the newspaper comics. He has a gun in his pick-up truck, which is parked out front. For one reason or another, he has not had an orgasm in two weeks, so he is horny, with a keen edge. His girlfriend, whom he truly loved, dumped him a month ago. In strolls a typical middle-aged couple with their attractive 20-year-old daughter. They are tourists from far away, in town briefly for a break from driving. They get drinks, take a table in front of the horny guy and, amidst their unheard conversation, the daughter laughs fetchingly, throwing her head back, her hair flowing, eyes sparkling. The horny guy fantasizes about his only chance for sex with the girl. He will attack the trio by chasing them in their car and running them off the road. He will kill the parents, rape the girl, kill her, then kill himself. Now, assign percentage points to each variation in this fantasist's mental picture, based on what you know about American men.

    a) Percentage of men who would fantasize about the girl at all
    b) Percentage of men who would leave violence out of their fantasy about the girl
    c) Percentage of men who would add a gruesome step by having the parents tied up to watch the rape, before killing them all and themselves
    d) Percentage of men who would leave out killing themselves
    e) Percentage of men who would kill the parents, rape and then abduct the girl to be used again before killing her, burying her and hoping to get away with it
    f) Percentage of men who would kill themselves because of the shame brought on to their families
    g) Percentage of men who, if the parents were not there, would actually chase and rape the girl, kill her, and either kill themselves or bury her and try to get away with it
    h) Percentage of men who would actually go through with the above scenario, as written

2) All of the parameters of Scenario 1 are in place, except that because our horny guy is an arsonist, an hour earlier he had set a fire that brought all

of local law enforcement to the location of the fire, so he knows that should he go through with his fantasy, there is no chance that he will be caught.

a) Assign percentages to (a) through (h) again, based on the horny guy's certainty that he will not get caught
b) Now compare the differences you have assigned in (1) vs. (2) to get a sense of how you view the American male's true primal nature. Think about how you arrived at these opinions

Next, give this quiz to your women friends and the men in your life to see how widely opinions vary. Be prepared for vigorous discussions. Even though the onus to abide by society's mores should be, in my estimation, almost completely on boys and men, American girls are trained to feel guilt over any sexual activity unless there is love motivating it. Forget about the desire to make another person feel good. One needs to move out of the United States to find a cultural milieu that promotes playful sex for its own sake. A friend of mine lost his virginity and then some after he joined the Peace Corps and went to Africa, where sinewy, ebony girls worked him over but good. Uptight American girls can be a big letdown after exposure to tribal delights. But the United States is still a relatively young commonwealth, so it may be expected to be backward in many respects, including sexual matters. It's no wonder prostitution is such big business in America. The United States of Repression will continue its role as the most violent first-world country until it comes to its collective senses and takes the fear and trembling out of sexual relations. And don't get me started on the problem of pedophile priests in this country. Again, it's a simple issue of men denying their true nature. Stupid, stupid, stupid religiosity. Note how these priests' repression dovetails nicely with kids' shame about being abused to form a perfectly sick symbiosis.

This applies to incest as well. One can only shudder at what must be the true scope of it, as boundless shame inhibits many if not most victims from opening up about their horrible experiences. The powerful exploiting the shame of the young may be at the root of most of what is wrong with this country. That, and hiding greed in the shadow of the American flag.

Still, today it makes more sense to write a manual for women who are faced with dating—or are married to—men who have had a prostatectomy. Does this practical approach take the romance out of the process of getting to know one another, that coyly incremental trading of smiles and laughter before that first kiss? Let's hope not. A users' manual could be introduced at an appropriately tender or funny moment to declare a man's vulnerability. Some women may prefer to feel their way along, so to speak, but given that most straight men are not big talkers, perhaps a manual is desirable. For you guys with wives or understanding girlfriends, feel free to glean what you will, but this is primarily addressed to the post-op men in their 50s and 60s who are widowed, divorced or otherwise single and seeking love or something like it. Herewith I make a stab at a very short users' manual for those who might want a summary of actions to be taken.

Sex with an Altered Me: A Users' Manual

Introduction: The Kindest Cut of All

Dear Romantic Partner:

Thank you for inviting me into your life. As we have discussed over the past few dates, I am nervous about intimacy. Although it may appear ridiculous, do not take my nervousness personally. It has nothing to do with you. I find you attractive, fun to be with, engaging in all respects. The cause of my nervousness is an operation I underwent some months/years ago, a prostatectomy, which I can either consider a blessing or a curse, depending on my mood. Understand that, generally, I hold on to a great deal of gratitude regarding the operation, as it got rid of the cancer that was in my prostate gland. The gland was removed so I no longer ejaculate any fluid. My orgasms are dry.

Step One: In the Mood

For decades I could count on my male equipment to respond quickly to arousal. Now, because the prostate is no longer there to regulate blood flow and trap blood in the erect penis, it is more difficult for me to get and maintain an erection. I use Viagra for short sessions or Cialis for a weekend in order to enjoy normal relations. Please be advised that once I may have been a proud jackhammer, but no longer. Today I bring a more varied toolset to bed, and I am a better lover for it. Patience, my dear.

Fundamental to my maintaining an erection is exercise, sufficient rest, lack of distractions, the right time and setting, and my belief that if you are patient with me, together we can establish a lasting bond. I want a long-term relationship and I want one with you. If that's not what you want, let me know as soon as you feel like telling me, but please, tell me before I am changed by your touch.

Step Two: It's All about You

You may have benefited from such experience previously, but in my case, understand that my mind is wired to please you first and foremost. My deepest sense of fulfillment is generated by your pleasure, not mine, despite spastic appearances to the contrary. After all, my sexual response is familiar to me, whereas yours is delightfully mysterious. Over the years, I have come to appreciate both the similarities and differences in the tone and texture of the female orgasm, and nothing is more intriguing. Even within the scope of one woman, climaxes vary enough in strength and nature that half a lifetime may not be enough to learn all there is to know about one woman's sexuality. But the quest to know another intimately is one of life's great joys and I wish to undertake that journey with you. Each woman is a galaxy of variation, womankind an inestimable universe. Would you please remove your clothes? Ah wait, I can help you with that.

Step Three: A Joy Ride

In this respect, when we first go to bed, I wish to employ the gentleman's imperative of pleasuring you first and thoroughly, before I am fully naked. Thus, in preparation of lovemaking, at some point I will have taken a Viagra, which takes about 20 minutes to kick in, giving me an appropriate interval to tend to your needs. Or, you may be done with me for now and flip on the House and Garden Channel.

It is known to (some) men that, should a woman be brought first to a deep and thorough orgasm, her mind will not only be cleared momentarily of whatever negative ideas she has about her partner, but her perception will be reconfigured to process the sight, smell and taste of his body favorably henceforth. I have learned the less-than-hard way to take my time, to build on one activity after another, tracing the calculus of a woman's psyche. Please understand also that one of the benefits of diminished hydraulic capacity is that the male mind compensates, much as a permanently blinded man adjusts to his reality by hearing and smelling more acutely. My interest in oral and manual investigations has increased greatly since my operation, without conscious effort on my part. Mother Nature does her thing to keep us interested in each other, come what may.

Step Four: Equipment Investigation

Once you have rested, panting and flushed, it may indeed be time to address my altered state, and what can be done about it. With the confidence of one who is certain he can finish what he starts, I kneel naked on the bed before your nude and satisfied form, to display my scarred belly and naughty bits (I love British tawdryisms). The eight-inch vertical scar running just to the side of and below my navel gives you some idea of the trauma inflicted during the operation. To begin the next phase of our experiment, for that's what these early times together may be, I suggest you employ my favorite lubricant and take my organ in one hand, to be gently massaged. If the Viagra has had time to open up the penile blood vessels, you will see and feel a swelling, signaling honest interest in you. Venture to use your other hand on my scrotum and especially where the scrotum meets the body, right at the point where the tendons converge, for here, my post-op body is very sensitive, sending urgent messages to the brain along the lines of "Hey, idiot, get busy with this woman, pronto!"

Step Five: When Two Become One

Your cooperative hands have done fine work to this point, and in some instances I will want you to finish me off this way so you can see me ride the pale horse, dryly, over the psychic cliff. But for our first few times together, we will make the best of the one-towel erection that represents the most I can muster at this point in recovery. In fact, it may be all I will ever regain in the tumescence department. We will make do with it, and coupling will not be that much different than if I were 70+ years old, with prostate intact. Say what you will about his stunted growth as a well-rounded person, but Hugh Hefner is still smiling, taking 20-year-olds to bed every night. So here, in our bed, hope and my penis spring anew, albeit with humbling limits. I truly hope you stick around.

Step Six: Rock 'n' Roll

You may prefer to be on top in the act of coitus, and trust me when I claim that all positions are fine, yet I am hesitant to remind you that blood flows downhill, so gravity now plays a major role in how I go about a successful encounter. This equates to the missionary position, or better yet, I keep my kneeling position. Standing works well for me, too, but in my 50s I'd rather be comfortable. The days of dropping trousers in an alley are over (I predict), unless of course, that's a kink of yours, in which case I'll get my keys and meet you behind the 7–Eleven in ten minutes. Kneeling is the best position for me to be able to maintain an erection, with missionary a close second. I should add that from time to time I can maintain a one-toweler while on my back if I hold the penis at the base between two splayed fingers, or if I use a rubber band, which inhibits the outflow of blood well enough for you to enjoy a brief straddling of the Organ of Longitude, as it is known throughout Eastern Europe.

Step Seven: Over the Top

On toward orgasm, Dear One, that we may become bonded as one, or at least as two having commenced something meaningful and fun. Most of the time, my orgasms will be dry, although I may sometimes release a small quantity of urine. Worry not, as urine is sterile, so simple post-act cleanup may be all that is rightly called for, unless you are hungering for more attention from me, in which case I will hear your signal for same by the sound of the shower coming on. As we lie in repose, and Henry Mancini strings waft in from somewhere, I am filled with gratitude once more, for you have accepted me for who I am today, with diminished erectile capacity and the other imperfections I bring to the party.

Step Eight: Last Tango in Pasadena

If you are one of those rare birds who prefers a sex act that is taboo in many quarters, my dear, you may have to get yourself another guy. I judge that such explorations require a minimum of three-towel strength erections, and that level of serviceability I have attained perhaps three or four times in the years since the operation, not often enough to perform a general repertoire. Such hardness surprised me, and I cannot account for those instances. Still, it doesn't happen often enough to adjust the menu. Perhaps a brisk spanking will suffice to excite the core of your id.

Step Nine: Oral Exam

Make no mistake, this activity is as mind-bending for me as any, and affirms your sexual powers. Until you have a clear comprehension of how my body reacts at orgasm, it is best to finish me with your hand, as I imagine urine tastes terrible. No matter how the end is achieved, the means will have been justified and I will stretch and then curl up, a happy puppy. I trust you need no encouragement along these lines. Oh, look! There's a diamond tennis bracelet under your pillow . . .

Step Ten: Resolution

Not to sound obsequious, but thank you, thank you for embracing my altered state! If merely months have passed since my surgery, the two nerve bundles in my groin that were saved by my competent doctor have yet to heal fully, so my orgasm may have scared you a bit in its intensity. It's as if there is no insulation on my wiring down there, and so it feels like my nerves are short-circuiting when I climax. In time, the sensations will return to normal. The lightning in my head scared me too, at first.

Men: So it goes. If you find yourself a woman who does not require porno-like jack-hammering, you should be fine in all respects once you return to one-towel status. Personally, I usually need Viagra to get there, but you may not. Still, a miracle drug is a miracle drug, so I'm not complaining. Good luck!

Nine

THE BIG O

There is a geometrical truth, made obvious by its definition, that parallel lines will never meet. Similarly, men and women will never understand each other fully, which is perhaps an equally immutable truth. Such is the power of gender difference. It sets us apart, forever, yet we must come together through attraction and compromise, to couple, have children and cat-herd them toward adulthood to perpetuate the species. To me, the social undeniability of this process is disturbing, but that's just me; I predict that in a thousand years, parenting will be a profession, not a biological given. Some people are great at it, others terrible, yet today society permits anyone to reproduce and take on the tough tasks of parenting. Did you know there are parents who send their infants though the belt-driven scanners at airports? And that, of course, is not the stupidest example of parental behavior in America. As young men and women, we look across at each other with wide-eyed wonder and longing, lust hard-edged, sanity taxed. If we're lucky, we learn over the years, and management of our differences becomes easier, even second nature. Yet the core mysteries will remain.

Certainly one of the most enjoyable aspects of heterosexual sex is guessing what the other gender is thinking and feeling, as their mental content comprises their closely held sexual identity. In other cultures, people are much freer to express themselves, even in most of Europe. (I have several tales of time I spent in Scandinavia, but my editor would cut them out.) Here in the United States, we still harbor remnants of post-Victorian repression, which some rationalize as modesty or something more self-righteous. In all contexts, however, women know that men love to ponder the details of a woman's sexual mindset and, for many men, myself included, one of the greatest rewards in intimacy is learning what makes a woman tick: her turn-ons (a very 1950s Playboy magazine type phrase, which I hate), and each little wrinkle in her sexual makeup. One thing men do know, however, is that women uniformly despise making fools of themselves in any sexual context, especially in public. Only the most secure of women can brush off sexually charged miscues in or out of the sack.

One of my favorite maxims, a tacit agreement among women, is that if by chance while they're walking their panties lose their elastic and slink to the ground, the proper response is to step out of them as gracefully as possible and continue on, without a look back or a change in expression. I have not been personally lucky enough to catch this phenomenon in real-time, but I do have some years left to witness it, according to my doctors. I am prepared to applaud cautiously, and from a distance. I am just as intrigued by the female of the species as ever, although my interest has shifted and evolved in a less animal direction. Today I can converse with an attractive woman without tapping my foot in an urgent, libidinal rhythm.

Based on a Philip Roth novel, there is a great film, *Elegy,* that opened in 2008. In it, Dennis Hopper's character George sheds advice like a snakeskin. Among George's observations is that gorgeous women, the so-called "10s" of the world, are invisible to most men; that is, the person under the finely wrought exterior cannot be truly seen. I'd never heard it expressed quite that way before, but it is very true. Men are content to speak and negotiate with the persona a given gorgeous woman has adopted and adapted to her ever-changing reality. Who she is may or may not ever become an issue for her pursuers, as the magical thinking attendant on acute desire obliterates reason.

This phenomenon can extend into marriage, as well as the shallow arrangements that are commonplace in L.A. I have had lunch with couples where the trophy wife is content to say hello and good-bye and that's it. The implication is that her physicality speaks louder and more eloquently than anything her mind might deliver via the spoken word. Truth be told, that precisely reflects the reality in some instances. Check out da Vinci's Mona Lisa. Her steady expression is worth evaluating as such silent, efficient communication. And of course, Los Angeles is the perfect town in which to see this cultural mechanism at work as, time after time, exquisite beauties are accorded deference whether they deserve it or not.

But some men cannot take the constraints that are mandated by society. It's a numbers game, like most every other aspect of life. One in a hundred or a thousand men break under the strain. They snap, to one degree or another. How many of us, behind closed doors, have raged against walls and other immovable objects in response to a woman's rejection or betrayal? Oftentimes, such rage is directed at ourselves, for feeling vulnerable, for feeling strongly about another person at all, for crying.

Other men relieve stress by acting out. Newspapers across the country routinely report guys who expose themselves at malls, or get nabbed for peeping late at night in housing developments. At 16, a buddy and I made feeble attempts to peek in cheerleaders' windows, but even when we could see in a bit, the blinds were always well-drawn, the lights quickly extinguished. There is a certain type of girl who lingers naked in front of windows, but we never managed to find one. My friend had a brilliant vision of us as the police arrived to arrest our enjoyment: "Two white asses disappearing over the hill." This is one of the most poignant images ever crafted, in my experience, and it's a shame my friend chose science as a career, rather than writing or some career involving women on the fringes of legality. He would have been so good at either, or both. This friend was the one who introduced me to both booze and the classic sex tome, *My Secret Life*. If I ever see him again, I will thank him for the introduction to the latter item. Also, his hand-carved wooden dildos and appreciation for the darkest porn films of the early 70s remain lodged in my memory as *noir* benchmarks of the male human condition.

Many over-stressed men who act out in public are, in all other aspects of their lives, normal. Those guys scare me. You know who they are, the sexual hypocrites of the world, exemplified by various pastors and priests who commit very human acts while condemning those just like themselves. Then there are guys who stand out, so to speak, from the crowd. Consider the case of Leonard Dickman, age 90 at the time of his alleged social experiment. As reported on the Web site thesmokinggun.com, in July 2007, Dickman was arrested for public indecency at an Ohio park. Forget for a moment that any variation in Cincinnati's behavioral landscape might be construed as cause for excitement. From the arresting officer's report on Dickman:

> Arrested was sitting in [2004 Kia] with his private parts exposed by raising the left leg of his shorts. Arrested later covered his privates and asked the arresting officer to watch as he moved his penis up and down without using his hands. Arrested also touched arresting officer's private parts.

The report also included details that put Dickman in a certain broad demographic: 5 feet, 8 inches, 129 pounds, wearing a tan shirt with an American flag, and tan shorts. In short, he is Everyman, albeit 90 and prone to airing it out in public. Dickman was, of course, innocent until proven guilty. I did not follow up on his case, though I am confident he got the slap on the wrist he desired. Send me $50 and I'll send you a Free Leonard Dickman t-shirt. (On second thought, make it $100. I have a busy schedule from now until I drop dead, though I trust I will outlast Dickman.)

What can we learn from this inspiring incident? One, Dickman expresses his gratitude for being alive in an unusual way. Two, Dickman may be lonely. Three, Dickman may have found the optimum mode for displaying mismanagement of the big O, which if one is not careful, may become the scourge of one's manhood. The big O comes on gradually, and once it gets hold of you, there is no turning back without recourse to hard drugs such as prescription testosterone.

No, I am not referring to orgasm, which might be defined as the physiological contingency supporting interaction between men and women. Rather, consider the *obsolagnium*, which Mr. Webster does not define in his pocketbook edition. Turn instead to the online *Grandiloquent Dictionary*, which offers "the lack of sexual desire that accompanies old age." Or, online again at Phrontistery ("thinking place"), which defines it as "waning sexual desire due to age." The former definition was probably penned by someone younger than the author of the latter. Equivocation in sexual matters becomes appealing as one's testicles become less active as surely as they trend earthward in life's last decades.

In 1999, when I was 46 with prostate cancer—panicked, depressed, and sitting in Dr. Kuyt's office—he'd had said that in a few years sex would not be as important to me because the urge would start to wane. He was trying to put my future in a context that he felt comfortable predicting, but I wasn't having it. Back then, I was still chronically blue, and sex with at least three-towel strength erections was key toward getting me through the days. When testosterone is still churning through your body with positive effect, it is daunting to hear that, not long in the future, your levels of that hormone are scheduled to lessen, ushering in diminished sexual desire. This helps explain why men in their 50s and 60s can be effective leaders and get so much work done; they are distracted by far fewer testicular storms.

Yet here it is some 10 years later and, sure enough, I have to embrace my own obsolagnium as the bellwether that it is. Now, male readers, I don't want you to panic, because, yes, I still want and enjoy sex. It's just that the urge is no longer a sharp and perpetual distraction. It's somewhat like the difference between being hungry at 8 P.M. when you haven't eaten all day vs. the hunger one feels anticipating dinner as the third meal of the day. In the former case, you are unlikely to think of anything but food until you eat, while in the latter case, if you skip dinner, you know you will wake up the next morning hungrier but still not famished. When I recall my youth, no sex for more than three days back then would drive me up the wall. Now, three weeks' deprivation produces a lesser effect. But what of the Dickmans of the world? Where are men like Dickman to go with their desires?

Leonard Dickman's wish for an authoritarian audience to the ups and downs of his withered penis was his way of declaring that he is not yet ready to go quietly into that cold, dark void where neither erections nor the twinges hinting at their potential exists. Dickman is expressing both his former capabilities and his fear of dying. He is an existentialist hero, one of the few, I venture, in Cincinnati. Though society may be appalled at his choice of behavior for expressing his feelings, I will stop just short of applauding him.

Those who know me pretty well can predict that if I am alive and ambulatory at 90, women of legal age loitering in the park might find themselves enduring a glimpse of my ancient equipment, as the pride I would summon then, should it move up and down at all—without hands—would be incalculable. In fact, I can foresee that until the stern arm of the law curtailed my activities, wandering to a nearby park to display my weathered apparatus might well be high on my morning agenda.

Ah, to be young again! Erections with an urgency beyond description, that feeling of need that renders all other thoughts insignificant. No food or water for days? No problem! No sexual release at least once a day? Put me in a straitjacket. Those were the days. Remember as a teenager when you would stew in your room, bored out of your mind? To me, this was nature's way of instructing us to lie down with a similarly bored girl and mindlessly copulate. As I see it, all boredom before age 40 has a sexual component. Certainly every episode of boredom I've ever experienced could have been cured by some sex, give or take. Then I'd take a nap and be good to go, just like the rest of the animal kingdom. Sadly, the culture condones sexual languor as a lifestyle only for the rich, condemning it in others.

My obsolagnium crept over me so slowly that I didn't notice it, until one day it dawned on me that sex had become more of a want than a need. It took perhaps three years for it to run its course, and now at 56 as I write these lines, my testosterone level seems to have leveled off, or plateaued, as doctors are fond of saying. No longer must I tend to the urge before anything else can get done. However many millions of years of evolutionary drive that were once ably represented by my eager "junk," as the younger generation is fond of calling the genitals, is now mostly a memory. My body now makes sexual requests, not demands. One would think that improved sanity would follow this transformation, and one would be right. I am a much calmer person now, and life is much easier to manage. For me in particular, the specter of drink looms less large as well, as booze and testosterone have a magnetic attraction in my personality.

Immediately you ask, is the trade-off worth it? Most of the time, yes, in my estimation, but I understand that my opinion about this issue is skewed by my having been clinically depressed for four decades. These days peace of mind is far more precious to me than anything else, perhaps because it is so rewarding in its unfamiliarity. Depression is an ill-defined prison, but a prison nonetheless, and it is an incredible relief to be sprung from it by both the aging and maturation processes (not the same thing, of course) and the antidepressant Lexapro. If ever there was a magic bullet to kill my gray moods, Lexapro is it. I must thank my dear friend and life coach E. Patrick Miller for both recommending it and for talking me into trying it. I doubt anyone else on earth could have done so.

However, I am still prone to occasional overwhelming and acute bouts of Neanderthalism that, predictably, are brought on by exposure to a beautiful woman. I consider these perfectly natural and perfectly intoxicating, and even though puberty for me was 43 years ago, I am never prepared for the feelings that accompany the swaying of a nubile woman's behind. Maybe I'm still crazy, but who's to say? I'm certainly not going to pay some shrink to tell me, so best to just soldier on with it.

For the reader, if you're not paired with one person after prostate surgery, I suggest you tread carefully if you're seeking long-term companionship. Find someone whose sex drive is at least somewhat in sync with yours. I cannot imagine dating the 25-year-old banshees who used to run me around the block back in the day. Luckily, stable women have an inherent mindset that appreciates serenity and stability in a man, for as childbearers and caretakers, they are wired to seek a safe partner in a consistently positive environment. Thus, most women should and will appreciate a calmer version of you, once the Big O sets in.

And what about sexual frequency in one's 50s, 60s, and 70s? In my mid-50s, once a week is enough, twice a week fine but not maintainable. In my case, this frequency is down from a peak of 10 times a week in my 30s and once a day in my 40s. These numbers reflect what my body naturally prompts, the incidence of orgasm that makes for a balanced human organism named John. But as John has intimated, he can go a couple of weeks without climaxing and not feel uncomfortable.

But what about the extremes, just for the record? In my 20s, one time in Florida (though not at band camp), there was a day and night with a pair of nutty sisters that produced four orgasms (all mine; theirs came in waves as continuous as in the nearby Atlantic) in a 24-hour period. That kind of effort would kill me today, and it would be a horrible psychic death indeed. Two a day is about it for me now, and I need a week's respite afterwards. Today, the second event in a sex session has to be coaxed out of the deep recesses of my mind, much as a black panther might be coaxed out of the upper reaches of a big tree in winter. Not so decades ago; then it was more like urging a fat spoiled housecat onto a kitchen table for another plate of milk.

Our female partners, as we celebrate, can go on and on alluringly, seemingly forever, but again, I am suggesting you find someone whose sexual wants and appetites match yours. Have you ever played golf with a zero-handicap woman golfer? Me neither. Needs are a trickier thing to manage, as denial of needs produces neuroses, and prompts secrets and unseemly behavior. Should you wish to play the field, by all means do what you can to enliven your experiments, as your apparatus will benefit from routine deployment. It is good for your postsurgical body to have erections routinely, lest you fall victim to the socially dreaded syndrome of diminished penile size. (Insert penis joke here, or a Zen *koan*, if you prefer.)

Yes, you read that right. For the first year or two after surgery, I experienced some shrinkage that was not remedied until I again made it a habit to give my variable appendage its marching orders. Not that I minded, but sometimes when you don't have a partner around, masturbation can be depressing. Not the best psychic direction for me. That feeling of numbing, double emptiness is not good.

My recall of Shakespeare is not splendid, but one would think obsolagnium would have merited mention by the great bard. Perhaps a line or two from Falstaff about the droop of graying years? There is something very spiritual about diminished capacity in this area, and there is a sense that, when it sets in, you are distanced somewhat from other mammalian creatures. One strolls the neighborhood and spies humping dogs with a wistful quality not unlike when one spots a porno magazine and is surprised that there is no urge to pick it up and flip through it. The lurid may now stay hidden, waiting for younger eyes to burn through such images.

That's life, you say? Perhaps so, but for the guy recovering from prostate surgery, feelings related to changing sexual ability are often amplified. One guy may see a pretty girl on the street and just sigh about days gone by—while another man who deeply senses he could not meet the shapely specimen's physical appetites might go into an emotional tailspin. It's not a good thing that the culture promotes sexual vitality as the most important measure of manhood, yet that's where all the advertising dollars go, to convince us all of the truth and wisdom of our clamorous culture. I know better myself, but sometimes I fall prey to the incessant multi-media messages and become resentful of younger men still with that virile cast about them. In my case, the related lack of semen and the lost native ability to reproduce does not faze me, as many years ago my father scared the drive to reproduce right out of me. Now it's just one less aspect of aging that could weigh on me but doesn't.

A little research into the Big O and one finds *obstipation* close by in the dictionary, which means constipation taken to the extent of complete blockage. I'll take obsolagnium every time. As the late, great Gilda Radner wrote, it's always something. It's just our bodies producing less testosterone, that natural drug that triggers all the fun and trouble. With 10 cancer-free years behind me, I have toyed with the idea of taking testosterone supplements, but I don't relish dragging my knuckles around again—better to let my physical circumstances settle in comfortably. However, if down the narrowing road my sex drive diminishes toward disinterest, then perhaps I will convene with Fred to buoy my organ with supplements. I don't intend to go out like Nelson Rockefeller, the late and former New York governor who died in the saddle, as it were, but I don't intend to lie down, without a fight, either. E-mail me in 10 years to see what I'm up to, and how I'm going about whatever it is I'm accomplishing in bed. If I don't answer you, assume the news is bad. If I send you a pic of a supermodel as a response, humor me and don't question my suggestion. I'll be doing the best that I can in either case.

So what to make of our lives once the sex drive has diminished to a more civilizing level? I find I have a lot more time to take on tasks that I have always put off before, among them writing this book, some screenplays and two other books I am working on along with this one. Give me those testosterone supplements and I will soon become distracted by any hot woman within range. Somebody somewhere said that if you're living your life right, you won't regret getting older. Oh, wait. I said that, at an A.A. meeting. I couldn't agree with myself more, as I now am more content, in my own screwy way, than I have ever been.

Many of my contemporaries, women mostly, live in morbid fear of each advancing day. Rightly or wrongly, I feel sorry for them. Approaching the end of one's mortal journey should be an enriching experience, not one filled with dread. It is never too late to take another, better path.

Some of us thrive only in the company of others, and living alone, or being alone, can be one of the trickiest propositions life throws at us. Perhaps your beloved has passed on and you are recovering from a prostatectomy with no one by your side, no one to talk to. If so, and you are moving forward anyway, you have my admiration for the courage it takes to keep from collapsing in the face of having been dealt another cruel blow on top of whichever hardship you have survived.

I cannot speak for women, but American men—well, you know what I think. When I lived in New York's Greenwich Village, I had a neighbor who was a retired Army officer. He was unfailingly polite, with an Asian girlfriend as quiet as he was. I recall trying to engage him in conversation one afternoon as we watched the battleship USS *Iowa* cruise ominously up the Hudson River. My neighbor was dressed head to toe in field dress fatigues, and managed only a smile in response to my stated appreciation for the immense warship, a most masculine relic of a time gone by. I cynically suggested that perhaps President Reagan had ordered the Navy to blast welfare recipients out of their tenements upriver. My neighbor smiled again, wryly, but said nothing. Shortly afterwards, on learning that our building was "going co-op," as the phrase goes, this veteran blew his head off rather than either move out or buy into the property collective. What or where were his inner resources? This guy had been a colonel in the service. Hadn't he learned anything about his own nature, enough to cope when life threw him a curveball? Or was he not at all accepting of the Big O, as he was in his mid-50s at the time?

I've recently learned the real circumstances around my maternal grandfather's suicide, and the subject of suicide has been on my mind, so I mention a few other such dire events to bring forth this idea: I believe that we all need to keep in mind that we are no good to anyone if we are not, first and foremost, kind to ourselves. This was one of the toughest lessons for me to learn. I had been so well trained to sacrifice my own happiness that I still don't think of it in terms of myself. I understand happiness when I see it in others. I feel that the best I can hope for is contentment or fulfillment. This is something of an absurdity, given how far I have come, but happiness to me is that mirage on a horizon forever out of reach. The only option is to keep driving in that direction or end the journey.

So I continue to peer through the metaphorical windshield and sally forth. Of course a good sex life is part of any worthwhile life journey, which is why I am so determined to get it in order. I am still working on it, as you can readily tell by my insistence on looking at every angle of sexual change that I encounter. Am I narcissistic for such unrelenting self-examination? Perhaps, but I make no apology, as all memoirs have an element of over-examination.

But forget about my midlife, post-op sexual travails for a moment. What do the experts have to say about that ol' obsolagnium that's got us in its spell? One matter they seem to agree on is that if you wish to make a firm, consistently good impression on your partner, make shared erections a habit. Writing in the August 18, 2008, edition of the *Los Angeles Times,* Regina Nuzzo states what might be obvious:

"Men who have erection problems tend not to have much sex, urologists noticed." Noticed? This is a woman writing, so I'll cut her some slack for that weak verb. Maybe she should have qualified it with "female urologists noticed." Thus, older men with erection problems may serve ourselves best by putting time aside to create erections on a regular schedule. The use it or lose it mantra applies.

The study cited by Nuzzo is based on questionnaires filled out by about 1,000 Finnish men aged 50–75, a group I daresay would respond honestly. People in Scandinavia consider sex to be part of their routine needs, rather than as a discrete activity fraught with taboos, repression and bigotry. And, yes, I've been there. The Finns in the study responded to questions about their sex lives, not including masturbation. Then the researchers asked these same men the same question five years later, thereby addressing obsolagnium, perhaps without mentioning it by name. Results included the fact that respondents who had sex at least once a week cut the incidence of erection problems in half. So why is it that the use it or lose it instruction works so well? The answer is oxygen, which, when the penis is purposefully stimulated, finds its way into the extremities of the penile tissues. Thus, in a man who has had prostate surgery, it is more likely to retain its size and shape if it is regularly swollen with oxygenated blood.

This procedure seems welcome enough, and certainly pleasant. Yet we may not have the urge for sex that we once had. For me, it has certainly felt odd to provoke an erection when I don't want one. My brain becomes confused, since once it prompted erections at the mere mention of the crack of dawn. The deep center of my id still clamors for sex without reasonable boundaries (in my case, this might mean two ruddy-cheeked Fox News reporters; for you, who knows?) but I am neither crazy enough to pursue these darker ideas, nor do I have the energy to fulfill them, most of the time. The taut-legged beauties at Fox News are spared my dirty old man predations, for now. Yet I am the last guy who'd wish to forego an exciting life. So, yet again, conundrums arise as frequently as my penis.

At the other extreme, if you demur from erections entirely, expect your penis to take on the aspect of scar tissue, no longer extendable for its intended mission. This is not my paranoia talking but rather Ms. Nuzzo, whose research I respect because the *L.A. Times*' editorial department vets its contributors quite well. So say you're 60 years old and haven't had sex for years. Then you meet the woman of your dreams, or even nightmares, and you have little to offer her other than a bent and withered old stump. Let us hope your charms and other assets are ample enough to offset any shortcoming stemming from sexual inactivity.

Perhaps I'm too strident in my concerns for a virile, older male population. But part of the purpose of this book is to avoid writing a follow up titled *I Told You So*. I suggest you stretch it in the shower, work up a semi-erection at least daily, and you'll be ready when opportunity knocks. Nuzzo notes that nature helps out with nocturnal erections, though she neglects to mention how she knows that. Acute investigative skills, no doubt.

(Side note: When writing a book, one does not always use all the research materials one has found along the way. In this case, I was about to begin quoting an author who includes among his beliefs a list of sexual myths attributable to the male. The problem is that I disagreed with the guy half the time, so I tossed aside all his writings as not in any way supporting my perspective. Such are the travails in writing about sex; there is often disagreement among those of us who offer opinions on the matter, even though our physical equipment works identically.)

Moving on to other resources, Jack Morin's 1996 book *The Erotic Mind* points out that sexual excitement may be reduced to a simple equation: attraction + obstacles = excitement. I tend to agree with that assertion, although when I was young, I think the equation that more accurately applied was: attraction x obstacles = excitement, implying more stress and neuroses when sexual drives are thwarted. I surely do not miss those pining times. Makes me wonder if the meaning of life is measured in how well we manage our disappointments. The word "no" coming from desired women's mouths has driven men to great and terrible acts since before we first earned the designation *Homo sapiens*. That being the case, is it human nature to want what we cannot have? I am not convinced. I think we learn to want things we cannot have as a distortion of, or amplifications of, normal or necessary basics such as food, sex, and honest companionship. However, I submit that our species is very amenable to learning any sexually oriented behavior that brings the genders together in order to meet nature's primary instruction. "A stiffening penis is extremely difficult to ignore," Morin writes, with an Oscar Wilde-like insight in *The Erotic Mind*. He does not mention ignored by whom—the owner of a given stiffening, or the beholder. Perspective regarding the penis is socially relevant.

And for that reason, we must be careful in submitting to cultural messages, many of which may serve our appetites, but at the expense of others. The case of JonBenét Ramsey comes to mind as a paradigm of culturally perverse messages resulting in horrific tragedy. Bad as the murder of the little girl was, I remain disappointed that her mother and father were not thoroughly vilified for sexualizing their daughter at such a young age. Tarting up a seven-year-old is to me the result of many poor choices, and thus terrible in the extreme. Is that primping and tarting up process what led to her murder? Was there a pedophile sitting in the audience of a pageant who took the parents' message to be aimed squarely at him? I would submit so. The case is still open, so we don't know and may never know who killed JonBenét, but I find what the Ramseys did to promote their little girl in pageants to be disgusting and revolting, and John Ramsey, the remaining parent, seems oblivious to his role in creating a gargoyle of a daughter who might have served as a poster child for—what? Nothing good.

That is an extreme example, easy to identify, that should be mythical, except it was all so sadly true. In more mundane lives, men recovering from prostate surgery have an endless stream of multi-media messages laden with sexual content to sift through, whether it's an eye-popping ad for Victoria's Secret or a raunchy song on the radio. These messages can serve to either warp us or reshape us into loving sexual beings. It is no simple matter to ignore the darker messages, nor is it easy to tread a corruption-free path. To paraphrase the late post-Jungian poet Greg Corso, our souls do indeed have shadows, in a very real psychological sense, and we must be vigilant lest we become confused by messages that can destroy us and others.

Lust wants, on some level, to achieve an autonomy that leads men to run amok. I have felt that tendency, and it was no small feat to curb my impulses. In my past, it has made perfect sense to me to be willing to sacrifice a pinky or little toe for one night with a particular object of my lust. Such is the pull of my opposites. And it is no anomaly that the United States has such a large prison population, as our cultural system of fast-paced messages, peer pressure to succeed, and the constant aura of temptation combine to create an atmosphere sure to beget men who snap or succumb to lust or addiction.

Helpful though such musings may be, there may still be a tremendous void there if you have not matured in such a way as to fill up your thinking hours with compensatory activity. I would expect you to throw this book across the room (spare the dog, not the cat, please) if I commenced recommending hobbies to you, so I won't. I will suggest that you find time for personal pursuits if you are the type of guy whose time is spent meeting the needs of others. Even though I derive joy from helping those I love, whether editing college papers or taking out the trash, I still find time to spend a day at the racetrack or, as always, to read, which both calms and excites my mind. In all things, I try to defer to virtue, but it is not always easy to identify virtue in its subtler forms. As a very smart friend of mine has said, man knows nothing of subtlety, nature everything.

If we are fortunate, in our waning years, romantic attachment (in my view a synthesis of lust and the need to surmount the fear of death by sharing experience with another human being) will not been lost even though the edge of our sexual need is dulled. For me, there is nothing like simply being in the moment, in a room, with my chosen lady. Words are so often superfluous. Minor perturbations in a shared space suffice to communicate our deep caring for each other. Her red plaid flannel robe diminishes nothing of her sex appeal, serving not only to keep her warm, but also to remind me that the daily routine I embrace answers most of the questions my heart poses today.

Thus, though sex occupies less of my time and attention lately, I don't stew about it, nor do I obsess over the option of taking testosterone supplements. Who knows, maybe one day I will opt to take that pharmaceutical plunge. In short, or rather in summary, please do not take your Big O as being a sign that you have one testicle in the grave. Take the attitude that serenity is to be welcomed whenever it finds you and that The Big O can be a huge help in finding consistent peace of mind. It's about time I wrap up my story, so let's get to the last chapter . . . of the book that is.

Ten

MADE WHOLE

Most of you reading this book realize that I've now enjoyed more than nine years of post-prostatectomy life by the time I wrote this final chapter. It has been, mostly, a rewarding journey, far more enriching than the future I envisioned back in October 1999 when I was staring at a hospital ceiling, waiting for my turn in the OR. I have been made whole again, by my doctor's experienced hands, by his wise counsel, by the support of those close to me, and by my activated belief in my ability to bounce back from adversity. True, there have been terribly bleak moments, but they have been brief, far between and part of my innermost life, which I find difficult to share. Those bleak moments are no more, I hasten to add. Today I have the same concerns as most people.

Overall, with this rambling narrative, I hope I have imparted to the reader the sense of gratitude that I trust I impart in person to those with whom I cross paths. And although it is obvious to us, it bears notice that, despite countless silly distractions, we all live in an age of fantastic scientific achievement, from which most of us benefit daily. I continue to be disturbed by the fact that there is no universal healthcare, as both doctor groups and HMO executives squawk about socialism at any hint that their incomes might be cut. And our government has heeded their concerns, quashing Hillary Clinton's attempts at a universal healthcare plan. Of course, the minute Wall Street needs a bailout, no problem, the Old Boys' Network rushes to action, lest that network fail and the old boys are left to struggle along with many millions of other Americans whose lives have been undone by a deregulated banking system. It has been clear to me for years, at least since the Charles Keating episode with Lincoln Savings Bank in the late 1980s, when the Old Boys' Network endeavored to steal many Americans' life savings, that the old boys were greedy to a serious fault. American businessmen in positions of the most power have proven time and again that they cannot be left to their own devices. Hence strict regulations should be put into place, as well as neutral, nonprofit-oriented regulators to police the banking systems.

What does the banking system have to do with prostate cancer? Well, if poor American men are to ever get proper treatment, universal healthcare will have to be instituted. There is no way we can afford that until the holes in our economic ship have been patched up. I don't think Obama can accomplish it until his second term, but I hope I'm wrong. Maybe he can do it in two or three years. We shall see.

With trillions of dollars slated to bail out various American businesses, why can't the guy who needs a PSA but can't afford the fee be bailed out as well? And if he needs an RP, why can't the supposedly greatest country in the world take care of its citizens first, before $600 billion a year is delivered to defense contractors to make instruments of death, which are deployed far from home in places where the local populations do not want us? George W. may have ducked the shoes at the December 2008 press conference in Iraq, but he will not duck history's appraisal of him. He did the best he could and I think for the most part his intentions were good. But he was not up to the job and set us back 10 years at least in foreign policy. Still, to his extreme discredit, he allowed Dick Cheney to enact his power-mad policies. It's a miracle Dick shot only one friend while in office. I will never understand how Cheney and his ilk escape the statutes of RICO laws that are supposed to protect us from organized crime. Again, don't get me started.

Now, perhaps, with a progressive, practical and very bright man, Barack Obama, at the helm of the Federal government, perhaps soon more men of stretched financial means will find it possible to get tested for prostate cancer and, more importantly, receive the surgery or other treatment they require. And perhaps improved educational programs and public service announcements will motivate men to see their doctors, after considering that indeed, prostate cancer can happen to them, and they may not experience symptoms until the disease is too advanced to cure. You will have gleaned from these pages that I find it abhorrent that America takes care of its defense contractors' needs before all of its citizens get medical help. American medical personnel are busy treating Iraqi wounds while the wounds of poor American children fester untreated. It is a revolting reality, unique in scope in the first world. I hope Obama does something responsible and lasting about this situation, and I believe he will.

Thankfully, the days are long gone when men whose cancer was contained in the prostate capsule underwent surgeries that effectively ended their erectile sex lives. Would I have written a book if that had been the result of my surgery? No, I would have retreated into private obscurity, as my spiritual well is not deep enough to thrive without erections. I knew a Californian named Joe who died a few years ago in his 90s. He had had the surgery before erectile nerves could be spared. He loved to joke with young women about how his enhanced oral abilities could compensate for his stilled appendage. Given Joe's lurid promises in the oral realm, I'm betting that women on Los Angeles' Westside are glad Joe is gone from the singles scene.

Nerve-sparing surgery is the norm today, for which we middle-aged and older men are grinning and grateful. I would wager that no books were written back then about sex lives with no erections. It is one thing to breathe a sigh of relief that one is still alive and healthy despite having no penetrative ability, quite another to maintain a positive attitude and focus long enough to complete a book about it. Certainly Joe would not have taken the time, even though he claimed to be a writer. And yet, even today, there are few books or articles written celebrating erectile capability postsurgery. I chalk this up to our ridiculous post-Victorianism, the depth and breadth of which is not quite sufficient to drive me out of the country.

As the reader can determine, I have no hang-ups about revealing what I can and cannot do with my favorite organ. Back in the day, an ex-girlfriend nicknamed me Captain Penetrato. I might suggest to her that that name overstates my needs and capabilities today. So be it. Sergeant Repertoire would suffice today. Every day I can either accept my physical limitations and find some peace of mind, or fight what is true and find fresh miseries. So here I am, glad to tell my story, as the near-decade interval between the kindest cut of all and today has been long enough for the leading edge of scientific method to have advanced again, radically, if you will.

For now is the time of robotics and laparoscopic techniques. My friend and surgeon, Dr. Fred Kuyt, no longer performs surgery, leaving those tasks to younger associates who are well trained in the latest laparoscopic advances. Cutting edge medicine in several surgical domains trends toward tiny incisions in which a robotically guided camera and cutting tools are inserted through to the target area.

From the procedure that has become the standard, LRPs (laparoscopic radical prostatectomies) are available at many top medical facilities. One can infer that much trial and error attended the development of this surgical improvement. The new standard is to cut five small portholes less than a half-inch long into the abdomen. Then, below the belly button, carbon dioxide gas is introduced to elevate the stomach wall away from the surgical site, giving the surgeon a better view and room to work with stick-like instruments. The improvement over traditional methods is significant with such keyhole-sized entry points: much less pain; less blood loss; a shorter recovery period; much less scarring; and a quicker return to normal routine. One would also think that the risk of infection would be lowered, but I have no information to that effect. Yet this is a tricky business, so men of a certain age should be doubly grateful that prostate issues do not come on suddenly, like problems of the appendix, or hernias. Coordinating the camera with the cutting instruments while viewing a video monitor, the modern surgeon performs an almost balletic procedure with the hands, but the results are that the cancer and the prostate are removed cleanly, almost bloodlessly.

And yet, although those seeking a surgical solution to prostate cancer no longer have to be cut wide open as I was, Fred Kuyt prefers the old school method in theory, as there is nothing, he judges, to replace the surgeon's open eyeball view of the operating area and the knowledge to be gained by feeling around the site of the procedure. Hands learn in a tactile dimension forever hidden from eyes. Still, with the most modern techniques, recovery time is shortened and there is almost no external, long-term evidence that surgery has taken place. Faced with the choice today, however, I would go old school RP again, long scar and weeks of diapers and all, based on Fred's judgment. Surely, around the country and the world, there will be many more "regular" RPs performed, as the latest robotic techniques will be slow to spread to less affluent regions. Once the U.S. embraces universal healthcare, poor men will be able to receive surgery, and many will likely undergo traditional RPs. I hope this book finds its way into such men's hands.

This comparison of the old and the new methods is not to minimize the short and long-term trauma of any prostate-removing procedure, no matter how it is performed, though of course I cannot speak firsthand about the latest techniques. Either way will slow you down big time, all but forcing you to take stock of your mortality and much of what men take for granted when they are younger, including near-instant, insistent erections.

Looking back at 1999, when I was diagnosed and endured the operation and early recovery, I realize that my sense of self was exploded into ragged psychic pieces, ostensibly not a welcome circumstance for someone who has felt alienated most of his life. But the good to come of psychic fragmentation stemmed from having an opportunity to examine my component parts separately, before they came together again, before I was made whole. Today, I can mingle in a roomful of attractive women and not feel "less than," a phrase describing low self-esteem that makes the rounds in A.A. If the topic comes up, I can describe to anyone what I have been through, without averting my eyes when I come to the parts that make me vulnerable. I can do this not because I have gotten better physically but rather because I have grown spiritually. I understand that if such information is shared honestly and forthrightly, I will trigger in the listener their mechanism for empathy and sympathy, for they too are heir to the maladies all humans may acquire.

I have counted on, with respect, the reader's certain knowledge that one day their own health will fail. Secure in this knowledge, we lean on, and in the best of circumstances, come to trust one another to advance toward that inevitability with dignity. For me, I take no psychic shortcuts. Sexuality is a touchstone of a mortality that is final and complete; when one does not believe in an afterlife, each intimate moment becomes important. As someone bent on gaining acceptance of my mortality without the crutch of religion, I learn from the great philosophers—Nietzsche (especially *All Too Human*), Kierkegaard, Mill, Wittgenstein, Lollobrigida, and others—who have expressed their thoughts so that the reasoning among us might identify with one another and bond accordingly. Their teachings, along with my knack for synthesizing and creating ideas of my own about the meaning of life and death, have created a truth and a belief system for me. I trust everyone has run some inner gauntlet of doubt to reach their own singular understanding. Perhaps the luckiest among us think about such matters not at all.

For me, an agnostic, my philosophy of gratitude and understanding finds its foundation in what the poet John Keats termed Negative Capability. For a high Romantic poet like Keats, as insightful a man as has lived on this earth, life is an excruciating balance of unpredictable love and pain, teetering on a fulcrum of risk. In this view, it is man's (not God's) sole responsibility to choose life-affirming actions for the benefit of himself and his fellows, even in the face of inevitable annihilation, while acknowledging that no God will ever affirm the goodness of such acts, either during life or after death. Is there a God? they ask. We answer with a resounding, if unsatisfying "we don't know," but we will act according to the Golden Rule anyway, because we have consciences that must be served if sanity is to reign on both a personal and public level. So the mandate is to soldier on even though we will never know if our actions are deemed good by a Creator. This perspective is too harsh for most to consider, let alone embrace, yet it is intellectually sound, given not what we know, but what we are equipped to know. Still, God may manifest itself in some way we do not, and cannot, understand. For me, any parameter of a God must survive man as, in cosmological terms, we have been around for merely a hiccup of time. As for size, it is daunting for most to contemplate that if the known universe were the size of the Earth, the Earth would be the size of an atom. They don't tell you that in Sunday school.

Until larger truths are manifested, I choose to leave the door unlocked for God and leave the light on, as it were. Indeed, I find it easier to contemplate no God at all over a God that sits back and watches manifold horrors on earth while choosing not to intervene. Could I ever pray to an entity that allowed the Holocaust, much less child incest, rape and disease, and the broad array of other calamities that befall good people? As a writer, it would be amusing to me to see so many human beings vest their lives in the religious writings of men who have crafted persuasive treatises to advance the deification of another man, except for the fact that men kill to defend their beliefs. Women, physically alluring to men and physically weaker, are put in an inferior role in all these treatises, because men resent women's sexual control over them. Religion exists to subjugate women, make no mistake about that, though I give substantial, albeit malignant credit to the writers whose elaborate work misleads so many. Women must be made to pay for their sexual control by being made subservient, supposedly by the word of man's God(s).

For what man among us has not been made to feel smaller by a woman's casual rejection? Thus is begotten the social order in most of the world, as the three desert religions vie for adherents. Women may get to say "no," but as compensation, men get to lord it over them because they are physically stronger. The threat of "no" is offset by the threat of physical harm. It boils down to that balance, with sex at the core of it. So, with some majority of people buying into these manipulations, I yearn to move not so much to Europe as to another planet, where more advanced beings take each other as they find them, without prejudice, and not what they hope to become, even in death. It's these yearnings that lead to the alienation I have spoken about throughout this book and that I fight to a greater or lesser extent. I might embrace my fellow man, no matter how stupid and fearful he is. Consider the Crusades, 9/11, Darfur, Mumbai in 2008, and the countless other atrocities man commits in defense of beliefs that live only so long as he does. What towering conceit to kill each other over varying, mutable conceptions of God! Still, the killing will continue, as In God We Trust. It says so, right on the money.

On a related note, psychological mumbo-jumbo does not fly far with me either, but I believe the solid scientific principles of both the Freudian and Jungian schools provide deep insights into who we are. Books like Jung's *The Symbolic Quest* have helped me greatly in gaining an understanding of the human condition. Freud on sex is genius, as he codified thinking and actions that have been prevalent for eons. Moreover, unlike Tom Cruise, I believe in the healing powers of prescription drugs that transform brain chemistry for the better. And I believe in the dialectical, talking method of psychic healing, as first practiced by the ancient Greeks and now in A.A. and its offshoots. It is important to talk about one's problems with both peers and professionals if one is to understand one's place in any human system, beginning with the relationship with oneself, and outward from there.

Have I exaggerated the importance of the antidepressant Lexapro in my life? I hope not. No longer do I dwell on suicide as an option, no longer do I perceive the world as unfolding in a series of gray images, no longer is it like climbing Everest to get out of bed and face the day. Clinical depression is a killer, both subtle and profound, both insidious and blunt in its effects, yet I have always been able to adopt a "tearless and unblinking eye" (to quote Robert Penn Warren) in considering issues larger than myself. Today, I am eager to meet each day on its own terms, to solve my problems with vigor, rigor, and dignity, and I can meet almost anyone halfway in any respect, in the spirit of compromise.

The very fact that you are a reader puts you, in my opinion, in select company, so perhaps I empathize more strongly with you. I appreciate anyone who reads, no matter what the material. I spent much of my young adult life searching for a hot, self-contained brunette who reads Voltaire on the toilet; perhaps, in the afterlife I am unlikely to encounter, I will find her. There is a quiet subculture of alienated people seeking other alienated people, as one might guess.

Or perhaps my near lifetime of alienation stems from the fact that God is a neo-con Republican, imperious and indifferent, sort of like Tom DeLay with unlimited power. Raised in a quasi-commie household, it goes against my grain to participate in the money-churning American culture as, in the truest sense of the word, money is what counts here. However, wealth and privilege can certainly be alluring when I am in, say, Monterey, California in August, where God most certainly keeps a summer cottage.

For me, the annual attractions of Monterey are the various car auctions and shows, and the town itself, a hybrid of San Francisco and Nantucket. It leaves little to be desired in terms of restaurants, shopping, sea breezes and nubile women, tanned and lithe. I go back as often as I can, healthy, erections at the ready and alienated no more. I cannot describe to someone who is innately personable what it is like to, for once, feel part of a larger community. It's like being paroled from an Edgar Allan Poe story into a Technicolor alternative world one had previously only heard about through dubious rumors. To give credit where credit is due, I must again mention Alcoholics Anonymous as having also been most instrumental in teaching me a sense of community. Also, as my mother passed in 2007, I have gotten closer to my sister and brother and their families. I play the role of eccentric brother and uncle very well.

From Los Angeles, on the drive north to Monterey, the coast road promotes a mind-bending mixture of awe and vertigo. There are sheer drops of several thousand feet to the rocks at the ocean's edge below, so I pick my spots to take in the view, vertigo being yet another minor issue for me. The scenery is magnificent, but I would not take that road southbound at night. There are a few short sections where the distance between you and the void is about two feet, with only a flimsy fence defining the chasm's lip. Monterey is but one exceptional destination I list among my favorites today, my loving lady by my side. She has been wonderful to me, and for me, over the many years we've been together. I remain uneasy, as one who feels he is undeserving of such love. Such are the echoes of an unsafe childhood. The damage in me is permanent.

Also on my mind for the reader is exercise. I must exhort you to exercise! Exercise plays a key role in my lifestyle, as at least once a week I work out to get the blood and endorphins circulating, and to iron out kinks in a 56-year-old body. If you do not exert yourself physically, yet are able to do so, I strongly urge you to take cardio walks with hand weights of at least five pounds each, for at least a mile. It will take you half an hour. If you are in early recovery after an RP, you may urinate a little from such exertion. Back off until continence returns. After a few months of just hand weights, add strap-on ankle weights of five pounds each and walk a brisk two miles. Then rest for two hours or nap, and go about your business. I guarantee it, if you are physically able to do that simple one-hour routine twice week, you'll feel great! It really, really works! Do this for as long as you are able, then cut back in distance and weights as the clock ticks into your 70s and 80s. Your quality of life will be much higher from these simple exercises. Eat right, three times a day, balanced meals of no more than you could hold in one hand. Drink water every day and eat fresh fruit a few times per week. You don't need any advice beyond that to live a long life. Oh, and try not to concern yourself with the stress incontinence that may accompany exercise, especially when working stomach muscles. A little leaking is part of the deal.

As for therapists, as a seasoned front-liner in the battle for happiness in a crazy world, I am a tough nut to crack, although I am certainly free with metaphors to throw around. Decades ago, one of my shrinks, the late and eminent Albert Ellis, spent hours with me, but it took only one phrase to cut through my defenses. "Don't catastrophize," he suggested. There was something about that phrase that stopped me cold, in the best way. Of course, he meant that I should "right-size" and prioritize adversity when serious things happened, not when my mind is creating stress because it demands that all problems be solved at once. That's how I once thought and felt, all of it because I was terrified by my father as a kid. Recovering from prostate cancer taught me that lining up one's problems and solving them one at a time was the way to go; I had to learn over the course of 40 years what comes naturally to most people. (Of course, no one warned me that, as a creative type, I will always have unsolved problems ahead of me, as that is the nature of putting ideas out into the world.)

And yet, for all of Ellis's experience and insightfulness, he did not comprehend that my brain chemistry was faulty. I know I hid the extent of my depression well, from most everyone. I saw Ellis in the early 1980s, but it was not until 2003 that my friend and therapist E. Patrick Miller convinced me to try Lexapro. Life has no longer taken an uphill course for me since then, though the bumps are certainly there. And because I am certain many men identify with my postsurgery journey, it became important for me to write this book. Yet at the risk of beating a cliché into the ground, if only one man's journey is made easier by these words, then I will have accomplished something. Such are the vagaries of telling one's story this way. I no longer want to have that specific voice, tangential of conscience, in my head, urging me to write and tell the truth about what it feels like to have an RP and recover from it. Even an alienated person like me will find a way to reach out, if properly motivated.

As I anticipate the last season of my four-season tour on the third planet from that ball of thermonuclear broth we call the sun, I have a t-shirt that reads: "Life Is Good." And indeed it is, even though I make my living in a solitary manner, pounding out books, screenplays, articles and consulting business emails, with the occasional phone call and in-person meeting thrown in to make me appear as if I relish human interaction.

Today, truth be told, I am curious about almost everyone I meet, on one level or another. Credit Lexapro to some degree, and the natural maturation process, but most importantly, I credit A.A. and myself, for the often unpleasant work I have done on myself, toward socializing myself. Only rarely do I fall prey to what Jack Morin, in *The Erotic Mind,* calls the love-lust split, that very stressful condition wherein one tends to become a beast in search of simple sexual gratification.

More likely, love and lust eclipse each other in a way that affirms both my role and my partner's. Yet it is important to admit that there is a dark part of me that misses the horny days of my youth, when irresponsible humping seemed to be the only worthwhile goal or activity. It doesn't take much to trigger a quick flash of that feeling: a suggestive glance on the street from a suitable woman will do it. The call of the wild does not cease as long as we are alive, though it should become indistinct and muted with time and maturity.

Those who have had, or are considering, radioactive seed treatments or cryogenic care for prostate cancer may be disappointed that I did not include much information about those alternative methods of treatment. This is deliberate, as I am a strict proponent of cutting out the cancer and putting it in a jar, as Dr. Bob Milch suggested to me back in 1999. I believe one has to take a stand on such things. If you want to investigate the option of freezing the cancer as treatment, a good place to start would be cryocarepca.org. Its proponents claim about a 90 percent effectiveness rate. If you want to look into seed radiation (brachytherapy), you can start at the American Brachytherapy Society's Web site, americanbrachy therapy.org. This treatment has become increasingly popular, as it leaves the patient with his prostate gland intact. As of 1992, only two percent of treated men chose brachytherapy, whereas by 1999, 36 percent chose it. It has become particularly popular in less advanced cases of the disease. For other forms of treatment, refer to cancer.org and prostatecancerfoundation.com. Prostate cancer has found a well-deserved and illuminated place in the culture of healing, and we should avail ourselves of as much information as we wish to acquire. For information junkies like me, massive amounts of information are not quite enough.

There is but one matter left to address. What of the future of prostate cancer treatments? I have read much about them and a few ideas stand out. Because prostate cancer has a strong genetic component, and because it originates where and how it does, I believe science will one day soon find a unique genetic marker that will lead to either an outright cure or a preventive magic bullet for those who are at high risk for the disease. Also, it makes sense to me that a more accurate diagnostic blood test will be developed that will definitively identify the disease at a very early stage, perhaps when only a few thousand cancer cells have formed.

Fresh on the pharmaceutical treatment front is abiraterone, which works by "starving" prostate cancer tumors. In a recent British study, up to 80 percent of patients treated with the experimental drug experienced tumor shrinkage. This is great news, but a half-measure, even if it is approved by the FDA. Disease management is one thing, a cure quite another. But certainly those suffering from a killer disease will take any help we can get. Experts are especially hopeful about abiraterone's efficacy for the 10 percent of men with prostate cancer who have the most aggressive and advanced tumors. Perhaps if a tumor can be shrunk, it can then be treated more thoroughly by other traditional treatments. The drug works by altering the "fuel," testosterone, which promotes cancer growth in the prostate gland and elsewhere in the body if the cancer has left the gland capsule. Nasty as the tumors are, they have the added diabolical aspect of creating their own testosterone, which researchers have only recently discovered.

To offset this self-sustaining element, abiraterone acetate blocks an enzyme critical to converting cholesterol to testosterone. In one dramatic instance, a retired 50-year-old London banker, with disease metastasized to his bones, experienced a 95 percent drop in PSA in an early clinical trial of the drug. According to *L.A. Times* staff writer Thomas Maugh II, the retired banker soon "stopped taking painkillers entirely and was able to resume a normal life." Wow. Read more about this drug at its patent holder's Web site, cougarbiotechnology.com. It is in clinical trials for breast cancer, also, which should not be a surprise, as breast cancer is the hormonally driven, mostly female analog to prostate cancer.

Even more recently, in February 2009, Thomas Maugh II reported in the *L.A. Times* that a study published in the journal *Nature* (lead author, Dr. Arul Chinnaiyan, University of Michigan, is working in the emerging field of metabolomics, which comprises the study of chemicals produced during metabolism) revealed that levels of sarcosine (a derivative of the amino acid glycine) in the male body, produced by prostate cancer tumors, may vary according to the aggressiveness of the tumor. A simple blood or urine test to reveal sarcosine levels could either augment the PSA, or in cases where a urologist strongly suspects PC, perhaps through a positive DRE, replace the PSA to determine the severity of the tumor. As part of the study, sarcosine added to tumors in lab dishes made them more aggressive, while blocking sarcosine made aggressive tumors less deadly. At last, there may now be a way to determine which PC patients should address their tumors immediately with surgery or radiation versus those who can afford to take a watchful waiting approach. Such advances will help drive down PC incidence and, more importantly, deaths from the disease. The latest U.S. numbers for 2008 indicate that 198,320 men were diagnosed with PC and 28,660 died of PC last year. These totals are down about 20 percent from recent years, a great improvement certainly, but nowhere near where we could be as a nation of more aware citizens.

Until such brighter times, we must remain determined and philanthropic in our efforts to bring more information and treatments to the forefront. If you are in Southern California in late September, I'd like to shake your hand. I can be found wandering the Cruisin' for a Cure car show, which you can read about at cruisinforacure.com. I hope to have a booth there on Saturday, September 29, 2009, with this book available, and perhaps in subsequent years as well. Please stop by and say hello. Another way of contacting me is through email. I welcome questions and comments, as long as they are constructive. I will be as prompt in responding as my schedule allows, so please be patient, especially if, like me, you have a wait problem. E-mail me at johnhallenborg@aol.com.

In the interests of being thorough, I must mention the following study. On March 18, 2009, the respected *New England Journal of Medicine* (nejm.org) published a survey: "Mortality Results from a Randomized Prostate Cancer Screening Trial." The report was authored by 24 MDs and PhDs. It is unclear if any of them were urologists, or if any of the male authors chose to have PSA tests themselves. The trial compared death rates of two groups: (1) a screening group of men administered annual PSA tests for six years. Eighty-five percent of 38,343 male U.S. subjects complied, aged 55–74 years, and (2) a usual care group of 38,350 same-aged men who were subjected to typical health care maintenance, which reflected PSA screening rates of 40–52 percent. That's right, in the usual care group, only about half the men in an advanced age bracket were given PSA tests, and in the screening group, for which a pointed effort was made to get men screened, 15 percent of the subjects did not care enough about their health to follow through with PSA testing. Pretty scary.

Without rehashing the results here, the gist of the trial's outcomes is that screening did not make much difference in death rates in follow-ups of subjects seven to 10 years after the study interval, 1993–2001. After seven years of follow up, the screening group revealed 2,820 patients with prostate cancer, and the usual care group revealed 2,322 patients with PC. Fifty men in the screening group died of PC, while 44 men in the usual care group died of the disease. Thus, one may to infer that PSA and DRE screenings are both ineffective. Moreover, when cancer is found, the results indicate that affected men are over-treated; that is, men suffer more from treatment (surgery, radiation, hormone therapy) than if the cancer had been ignored. These results are merely a summary of an extensive report that is worth reading if one is so inclined.

The author and Dr. Fred Kuyt find the methodology of these trials to be disturbing. Why was the youngest person tested aged 55? That's too old. Why wasn't the differentiation in screening rates, 85 percent versus 40–52 percent, stressed more, as the two groups were not that clinically partitioned, as is suggested? That is the least of it. When I asked Fred if he had read the study, he replied in an email: "I've read it, am unhappy with such a publication by nonurologists in such a highly thought of and prestigious journal. I am not brave enough to stop screening my patients. That's because I cannot reconcile the results within my practice."

So what does being "made whole" mean for me, exactly, and what could it mean for you? It means that when I'm not writing about the disease and its treatment, I go about my business with no sense of debilitation. It means that the fact that I had major surgery years ago is as much an event in my past as is the knee rebuilding I had in my 20s. It is a milestone, yes, but not one I collide with time and again. Are my erections less firm? Yes, they are, but I have compensated in the ways described herein.

I am made whole because my personality is more integrated than it has ever been, and it continues to integrate more fully day by day, as my spiritual, personal, business and creative selves integrate well. Being made whole means I am available to others, to help them, give advice, and provide a shoulder to lean or cry on.

It means I am a great listener, tuned in to nuances of the spoken and unspoken. It means I have become a useful member of my community at the local, regional, and national levels. It means I have, despite my several infirmities and mitigating defects of character, become a good man. This I take to be the most desirable goal I could attain. If I am indeed there, or achieve "good man" status someday, in the estimation of my peers and those I love and who love me, I mean to maintain that auspicious station, faults and all.

One last bit of advice. As we move into our 70s and 80s, we tend to lose interest in sex. Nonetheless, we might want to keep our Viagra and Cialis prescriptions active, as a tiny amount once a day could help keep the heart pumping and one's shoes dry. Find each other, find love, find fulfillment. Enjoy yourselves, my brothers and sisters, and thank you for your kind attention to my story.

BIBLIOGRAPHY

Morin, Jack. *The Erotic Mind*. New York: HarperCollins, 1995.

Oesterling, Joseph, M.D., and Mark Moyad, MPH. *The ABCs of Prostate Cancer*. Lanham, MD: Madison Books, 1997.

Walsh, Patrick C., M.D., and Janet F. Worthington. *The Prostate: A Guide for Men and the Women Who Love Them*. New York: Warner Books, 1997.

INDEX

About the Author

JOHN C. HALLENBORG has been a freelance business journalist for more than 20 years. Currently he is working on two novels and two nonfiction books, one about genius and another about a former CIA operative's Cold War activities. John lives on the beach in Los Angeles.

www.ingramcontent.com/pod-product-compliance
Ingram Content Group UK Ltd.
Pitfield, Milton Keynes, MK11 3LW, UK
UKHW020821290926
15470UKWH00003B/1294

9 780275 981358